Microbiome Me

ISBN: 9781794050945

January 2019

By Peter V. Radatti

10 9 8 7 6 5 4 3 2 1

<u>Copyright Notice and Editions</u>

"Microbiome You" is the second volume of the Dietary Fiber Series by the same author. The first book in the series is: "Dietary Fiber, Essential to the Human Microbiome and Health". ISBN-13: 978-1545015421

Table of Contents

Preface

This is the second book in the dietary fiber series. Each book stands alone but each adds to the total knowledge imparted. Each book is a little different with a slightly different but related topic. There is some duplication from the first book where I felt it necessary. See the copyright notice page for details of the first book.

Keep in mind that I am not a medical doctor, and this is not a medical book. Please read the disclaimer to get a better idea. This book is intended as educational only. There are many footnotes to websites where you can learn more on almost anything mentioned in this book.

The controversy in this book is that I point a finger to a culprit who is responsible for the dire conditions we all find ourselves in. Talking truth to power is not a healthy thing to do but in this case the US Congress is used to being called on the carpet and, it is not the current Congress's fault. It is past Congresses that did us. The current Congress has a rare opportunity to help us by learning about the Microbiome and changing laws to remove poisons and insure the supplementation of our foods with critical mixed dietary fiber.

Instead of fighting over universal healthcare they could be providing universal health. Medical expenses could be so low that who paid became irrelevant. If they won't do it then vote with your money and avoid dangerous foods and buy foods containing dietary fiber to the extent you can.

I refer to a movie, "That Sugar Film" in this book. It is very well worth buying. If you decide to go on a weight loss diet, then watch this film every week. It will give you the willpower needed. There is a second film that you may also want to purchase, "The Magic Pill", subtitled, "Food Is Medicine" by Peter Evans. Both films have websites.

The diet plan at the end of this book is a work in progress. I am on the diet myself and I am learning more about what I can and cannot do every day. I am surprised by how forgiving this diet can be. There are a lot of books and websites that describe pescatarian diets. Some describe it as a vegetarian diet. It is not. In any case as I have more experience, I will publish my weight loss results.

The title of this book is an insider joke. One of my favorite modern movies is, "Despicable Me" so I shortened the title of this book to "Microbiome Me". It also allows me to refer to the book as M2.

Finally, this book has been professionally fact-checked and reviewed by both a copy-writer and several lay-persons prior to publication. I refuse to waste your time or mislead you in any way with this work. Having said that, thank you for reading my book!

Peter Radatti
February 2019

Postscript: Just as this book was finished Dr. Dean Howell, ND provided a bonus chapter on his experience rebuilding his microbiome. His website is http://drdeanhowell.com/

If you like this book, please leave a review.

Right now, about 1 in every 350 purchasers of my books leave reviews.

They are truly gold to an author and help motivate us. Please consider leaving a positive review.

If you hate my books, please don't tell anyone. That's a joke! Anyone who hates my books will tell everyone and generally loudly.

Thank you,

Pete

Dedication

This book is dedicated to my parents, Marie D. Radatti and Vincent J. Radatti, and to my Aunts and Uncles and friends. These people made me who I am. To the divine spirit who made all possible, including the miracle of life.

Additional Thanks to My Patron Saints: Saint Jude Thaddeus, Mother Mary, and Saint Rita.

Thank you to my editor, Barbara Higgins. You can learn about her fantasy books at her author's page of: amazon.com/kindle-dbs/entity/author/ B07HVN92CY

I am fond of her Sherlock Homes book, "A Most Dangerous Prey"

The cover artwork was licensed from istockphoto.com

All trademarks are the trademarks of their respective owners.

Finally, this book is dedicated to you, my readers. Without you this book is nothing more than words rotting away on a shelf. With you this book is knowledge.

<u>DISCLAIMER</u>

This book is being presented to the reader for informational purposes only. It is meant to assist the general public in learning about dietary fiber and the microbiome. Nothing in this book is intended to serve as legal, medical, scientific, or spiritual advice in *any* matter; it is for educational purposes *only*. Each reader will and must draw their own unique conclusions about the material presented, and if the reader attempts to implement said material, that is entirely their responsibility.

The information provided in this book is designed to provide helpful information on the subjects discussed. It is *not* meant to be used, nor *should* it be used, to diagnose or treat any medical condition; this is the sole purview of your physician. The publisher and author are *not* responsible for any specific health or allergic conditions that may require medical supervision and are not liable for any damages or negative consequences from any treatment, action, application, or preparation to any person reading or following the information in this book. References are provided for informational purposes only and do *not* constitute endorsement of any websites or other sources. Readers should be aware that the websites listed in this book may change.

This book is not intended as a substitute for the medical advice of physicians. The reader should regularly consult a physician in matters relating to his/her health and, in particular, with respect to any symptoms that may require diagnosis or medical attention. If you think you may be suffering from any medical condition, you should seek immediate medical attention. You should never delay seeking medical advice, disregard medical advice, or discontinue medical treatment because of any information in this book.

Without prejudice to the generality of the foregoing paragraph, we do not represent, warrant, undertake or guarantee:

1. that the information in the book is correct, accurate, complete or non-misleading;

2. that the use of the guidance in the book will lead to any particular outcome or result; or

3. in particular, that by using the guidance in the book you will have any result whatsoever.

If a section of this disclaimer is determined by any court or other competent authority to be unlawful and/or unenforceable, the other sections of this disclaimer continue in effect. If any unlawful and/or unenforceable section would be lawful or enforceable if part of it were deleted, that part will be deemed to be deleted, and the rest of the section will continue in effect.

Nothing in this book should be considered medical advice. For the treatment of any medical condition, you must seek the advice of a trained, medical doctor. This paper is *not* written with any specific products in mind but, rather, as a research of what is currently known about dietary fiber in general regarding nutrition.

The Microbiome

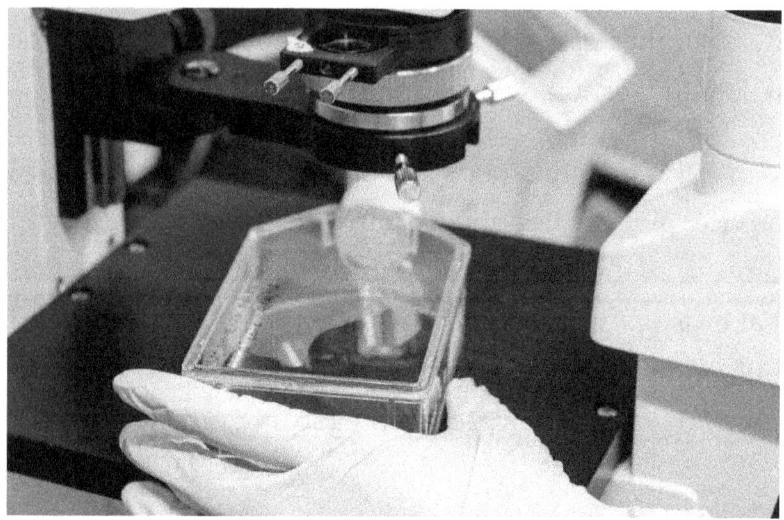

This book is about the Microbiome and how it helps to create who you are. There is more than just a gut-brain connection. There is a gut microbiome to brain stem connection via the Vargas Nerve and via blood chemistry.

I believe in the next dozen years we will learn more about how to affect the microbiome in order to improve health and clarity of mind. It is already known that certain bacteria that can affect humans make us seek out high risks, still others can make us obese. What other marvels will medical science discover!

Another interesting fact is that you don't have one microbiome, you have many. Nothing is a one size fits all when talking about microbiomes. This book deals mostly with the microbiome of the gut, one of the most important, however every part of your body has its own unique microbiome. As an example, there are multiple microbiomes of the face. The outside of your nose is different from the microbiome of the cheeks, forehead and eyelashes all of which may be different from each other. Every organ has a different microbiome. The concept from wine of Terroir[1] may also hold true for microbiomes.

---

[1] https://winefolly.com/tutorial/terroir-definition-for-wine/

The Role of the Physician

This book is not intended as a substitute for the medical advice of physicians. The reader should regularly consult a physician in matters relating to his/her health and, in particular, with respect to any symptoms that may require diagnosis or medical attention. If you think you may be suffering from any medical condition, you should seek immediate medical attention. You should never delay seeking medical advice, disregard medical advice, or discontinue medical treatment because of information in this book.

If you intend to follow the diet suggested in this book you must consult a medical doctor prior to initiating the diet. Failure to do so may lead to serious problems.

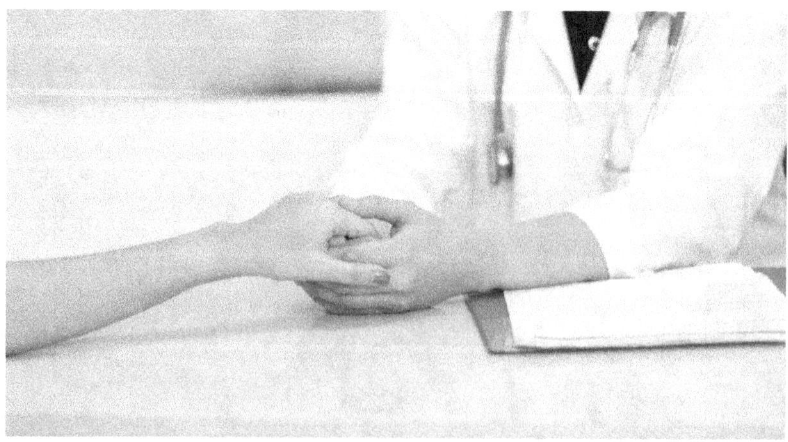

Fair Disclosure

I own a business that manufactures foods based on high fiber formulas. Radatti Foods, LLC is a start-up that is restarting manufacturing in 2019. It exists because former customers crowd sourced the funds necessary to bring the company back to life. (www.radattifoods.com). It was not something I expected or even wanted to do! My friends kept asking me to bring the products back and I kept telling them no. When they asked what I would need to bring the company back I replied, "startup expenses". They found it! Surprised me. Next time, I won't answer.

I did not write this book to enhance the company or sell products. I wrote this book for the same reason that I started the company, which is that I am totally fascinated with the subject of dietary fiber, the microbiome, and how they interact to create us and sustain our health. This book was me, pulling information together that I learned from many sources, while attempting to generate an easy-to-understand explanation of how it all works. I have only partly succeeded, but this is my best attempt to date. This field of study is vast and only just starting. We haven't even reached the low hanging fruit yet.

In addition, it is my opinion that if the knowledge in this book were common within the medical community, that multiple people I loved would still be alive today.

Radatti Foods does not believe it is easy to change dietary habits that we develop over a lifetime. Unfortunately, those habits have been formed by governmental interference and industry. We have gotten used to taking highly processed and sugar laden foods as normal and desirable. Radatti Foods believes that instead of changing people to desire beneficial foods we should change the desired foods to be beneficial high-quality foods. We do this by blending multiple dietary fibers until we arrive at something that is acceptable and healthy. Apparently, that is a unique approach.

This is an educational and opinion document, not a sales pitch. I don't even soft pitch products that I manufacture here. If you want to know more, you will have to visit the website and look for yourself. Be warned that Radatti Foods does not retail or wholesale and finding product may be hard. That will either self-correct or become even harder in the future as the company succeeds or fails.

Radatti Foods, LLC.

http:\ \ www.radattifoods.com

The sole distributor for Radatti Foods is:

The Essence of Life,

451 6th Avenue

Brooklyn, NY. 11215.

Phone: +1 (718) 788-8783.

A Wonder Food?

I also want to post a warning here. Many people tend to read a book like this and jump off the deep end, believing that the subject matter is a "cure" for what ails them and is some new "wonder drug/food". This would be a mistake. Dietary fiber is important, and I believe it is critical to health, but it is *not* a cure all! There is no such thing as a cure-all.

If dietary fiber has a large effect on the health of our population, which I believe is true, it is only because it has been missing in our modern diets. If we were still eating like our ancestors were, or even the way we ate in the 1950's, this book wouldn't have reason to exist.

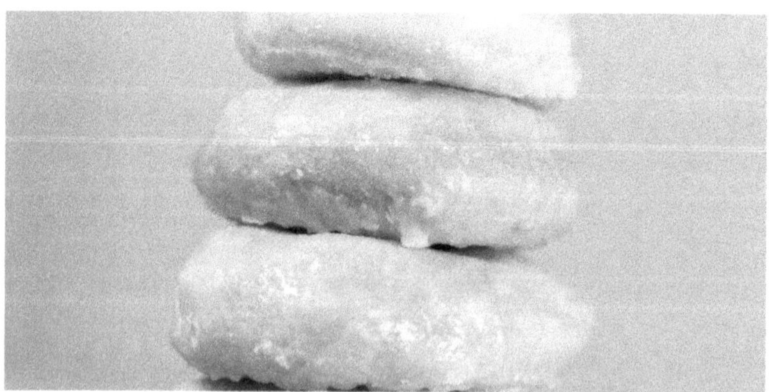

Sugar may be a wonder food in we can wonder how something that tastes so good is so bad for us. On the other hand, sugar has been around a long time and very few people were fat in the near past. What is new is the amount of hidden sugar we are eating, and the new man-made sugar concentrate high fructose syrup.

Finally, discuss with your medical doctor or pharmacist if you can take supplements or medication concurrently with dietary fiber. Sometimes you cannot!

<u>Your Microbiome is You</u>

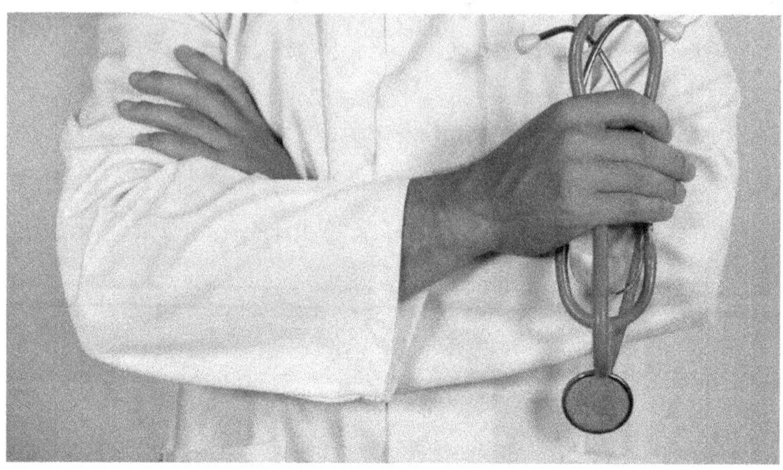

You are about to enter the Twilight Zone[2], The Outer Limits[3] and Alice's Wonderland[4] all while remaining firmly here.

You see, the world is not what you think it is. YOU are not what you think you are. Reality is real, but we just don't know it. We are only getting to the point that we understand we don't know what we don't know.

---

[2]   Registered Trademark of CBS Broadcasting.

[3]   Registered Trademark of METRO-GOLDWYN-MAYER STUDIOS INC.

[4]   Registered Trademark of DISNEY ENTERPRISES, INC.

This book will open the door just a little bit. It is going to concentrate on you and what you are. You will be surprised because you are not what you always believed yourself to be, and yet you are. This new knowledge is old knowledge but now we know why. This knowledge will give you the power to edit yourself. You can make yourself into a better you. A healthier, clearer thinking, quicker, perhaps even physically younger you.[5] All this is possible within you right now and it won't cost you any money, you won't have to learn esoteric mental controls, rely upon external forces, expensive herbals, drugs or gene editing. Yet, you will have a greater control over your gene expression[6] than you could ever believe. All by modifying something that you do anyway, every day of the week.

This will explain some of your thought processes and where some self-destructive thoughts may be coming from. You will truly understand the very old expression, "I had a gut feeling". There is a direct connection between your brain, your gut and your microbiome which helps you to think.

---

[5] Body age, not chronological age.

[6] Gene expression is what determines which parts of the DNA to execute and which parts remain dormant

You will learn why some self-destructive eating habits are very hard to stop, why weight loss is hard to do and a program that will work. It will still be very hard to do but it will work.

Finally, you will learn about your microbiome, how it affects you and how to heal it using dietary fiber.

I would like you to watch a few videos. These videos are associated with a book that I wrote called, "Dietary Fiber: Essential to The Human Microbiome and Health"[7] and a YouTube video. The videos and links as well as any updates can be found at:

http://www.radatti.com/books/MicrobiomeMe

The DVD videos and the books are available for purchase on amazon.com.

What does any of this have to do with what I was saying? I will explain. Let's start with the basics. <u>What</u> are you? Not who are you but what are you. Most people would answer I am a human. I am going to reply that is not true. YOU ARE NOT A HUMAN by the most

---

[7] https://www.amazon.com/Dietary-Fiber-Essential-Microbiome-Health-ebook/dp/B07DV2ZF8W/ref=sr_1_2?ie=UTF8&qid=1547047202&sr=8-2&keywords=radatti

common standard of what is considered to be human. Don't worry, nothing has changed but the standard of what we consider to be human is wrong. We believe that a human is a being that is composed primarily of human cells. That are cells that contain human DNA and RNA.

Science now knows this to not be true. Your body is only 10% human by cell count. Of that 10% a significant part of human cells is not human.[8]

What are the non-human parts of your body? Simply put it is bacteria and fungus. Yes, 90% of your body is and always has been and always will be bacteria and fungus. Don't let this upset you, nothing about you has changed. This has always been true.

Let's examine the 10% of you that is human. I define this as the parts where human DNA rules. Even this is not factual. This human part of you is still significantly bacterial. The mitochondria are the power plants that runs all human cells. They generate the ATP (Adenosine Triphosphate) chemical energy that is critical for human life to exist. No ATP equals no life. There are thousands of mitochondria in each cell and the mitochondria share no DNA with humans. Their DNA and RNA are bacterial.

---

[8]   Note, this is cell count, not cell weight.

For the sake of argument, lets reduce thousands of mitochondria to just one thousand per human cell. So, 1/1000 of human cells are human by cell count. Therefor 0.001% of your human cells are human. Remember that 90% of your body is totally bacterial? Now let's add in the real numbers.

90% bacterial + 9.9999% mitochondria = 99.999%[9] of your body is non-human <u>by cell count</u>.[10]

Let me allow this to sink in for a moment.

99.999% of your body is not human. Less than 1% is human.

Did I just run a train through your mind? I hope so but that is not the significant take away. Here it is; all medicine, all health information, all processed foods are geared toward the human parts of you. It ignores 99.999% of your body. No wonder we are so unhealthy as a nation.

It is worse than that. We are actively attempting to kill off the 99.999% of your body that keeps you alive and healthy!

---

[9] This math is a little wonky but basically as a matter of information correct.

[10] This is cell count, not cell weight. Human cells out weight bacterial cells by a substantial amount.

Let me repeat that then explain. We are actively attempting to kill off the 99.999% of your body that keeps you alive and healthy.

Things you do every day, products that you use every day, chemicals that you are not even aware of consuming, but are, these are trying to actively kill off bacteria and you are paying for this privilege.

<u>Water</u>

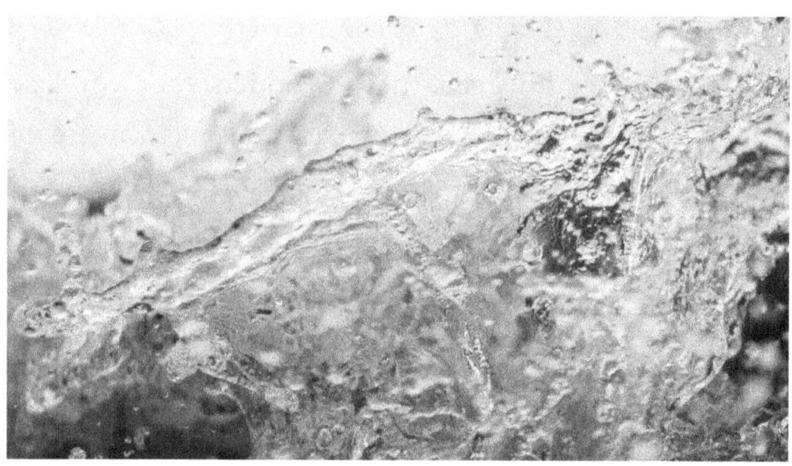

Let's start with some basics.

Tap water in the United States normally contains Chlorine. Chlorine is the gold standard because it kills off all bacteria and it is inexpensive. Not all countries still use Chlorine.[11] France mainly uses ozone. Italy and Germany use ozone or chlorine dioxide as a disinfectant. If you can smell the chlorine in your tap water, then you are ingesting chlorine when you drink it. What do you think the chlorine does inside of your body? It continues to disinfect. It kills bacteria.

---

[11] https://www.lenntech.com/processes/disinfection/reg
ulation-eu/eu-water-disinfection-regulation.htm

Bottled water may not be the answer. Many famous brands of bottled water are nothing more than tap water that has been purified and flavored with minerals.[12] Some bottled water is disinfected using Ultra Violet radiation or filtration or distillation. Bottled water has been found to contain phthalates[13], mold, microbes, benzene, trihalomethanes, even arsenic. Phthalates are known to damage the liver, kidneys, lungs, and reproductive system, especially male testes, according to animal studies.[14] You and I are the human studies. Even if you buy BPA-free plastic bottles there are other chemicals which can seep out if exposed to heat (warehouse, home or car trunk) or sit around for a long time. Some of these chemicals are possible endocrine (hormonal) disruptors. So bottled water may be worse for you than tap water and yet it costs over 1000% more than tap water. If your water contains fluoride, then consider only drinking and cooking with bottled water.

---

[12] https://www.mindbodygreen.com/0-11193/7-reasons-to-never-drink-bottled-water-again.html

[13] Phthalates are chemicals used to make plastics soft, like in water bottles.

[14] https://noharm-uscanada.org/issues/us-canada/phthalates-and-dehp

<u>Disinfectant Soaps</u>

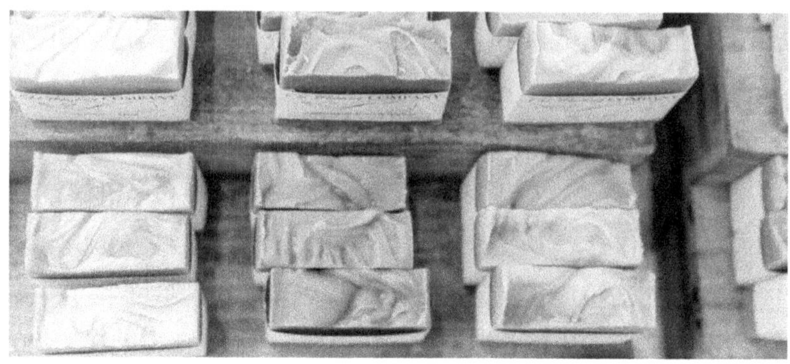

While we are on the topic of water lets discuss a related topic. Soap. In fact, there are two different things we call soap. The first is soap. It is made from fats/oils and Lye. The other things we call soap are detergents. Detergents are not soap and work by lowering the surface tension of water so that dirt and oils can go into solution easier. Many soaps are made from bleached rancid oils. High quality soaps are made from coconut oil, palm oil or animal fats that do not go rancid as easily. None of these are serious problems.

What is a serious problem are antibacterial disinfectant soaps. It is generally believed that anything you put on your skin is absorbed within 26 seconds.[15]

---

[15] https://www.ursamajorvt.com/blogs/the-blog-cabin/37974081-how-do-toxics-enter-our-bodies

There is good reason to believe this and three pathways have been identified, intra-cellular, inter-cellular, and trans-appendageal. Antibacterial soaps kill the beneficial bacteria on your skin that not only helps protect you from external infection but helps to keep your skin youthful and flexible. Once absorbed the antibacterial chemicals continue to kill off the bacteria in your body. Is this a problem? Yes. Ask a plumber what the effect of antibacterial soaps are on your drains. He will tell you that it kills off the good bacteria that keeps your drains clean. When people switch to antibacterial soaps, they eventually need to have a plumber run a drain cleaner to open the drain. Could this happen inside of you? Does your body have the equivalent of clean water lines (arteries) and drains (veins)? What about your digestive track?

The United Stated Food and Drug Administration issued a final ruling on September 2, 2016 removing 19 specific active ingredients including the most common triclosan and triclocarban from consumer antiseptic wash products.[16]

---

[16] https://www.fda.gov/newsevents/newsroom/press announcements/ucm517478.htm

Soaps are not the only problem. Personal care products can be dangerous. An example is lipstick. Some lipsticks contain lead.[17] Apply lipstick several times per day and absorb several times the amount of heavy metals. Fragrance may contain phthalates which can be inhaled. Phthalates are the same class of dangerous chemicals we spoke about earlier in plastic water bottles. This is just the beginning. Anything that you put on your skin you are putting in your body. That includes things that you put on accidentally like gasoline or weed killer. A general rule of thumb is if you can't eat it don't put it on your skin.

What do people in other cultures use instead of bath soaps? Older Korean men sometimes use loofah(s) on a stick but here in the USA some use low cost green scrubbies which are normally used for dish washing.

Don't rub hard if you decide to use these, use long gentle stokes and buy the softest ones you can find. The scrubbies the dollar stores sell 10 for $1 seem to work for me. Before you decide this is crazy you should consider that this is basically a cheap version of the

---

17   https://www.ursamajorvt.com/blogs/the-blog-cabin/37974081-how-do-toxics-enter-our-bodies

Korean Exfoliating Mitt recommend by Vogue magazine.[18] I like to use these in the shower.

---

[18] https://www.vogue.com/article/korean-exfoliating-wash-cloth-mitt-dermasuri

Laundry Detergent

There are problems with some popular laundry detergents. It turns out that some detergents leave residue on the clothes which is then absorbed by the skin.

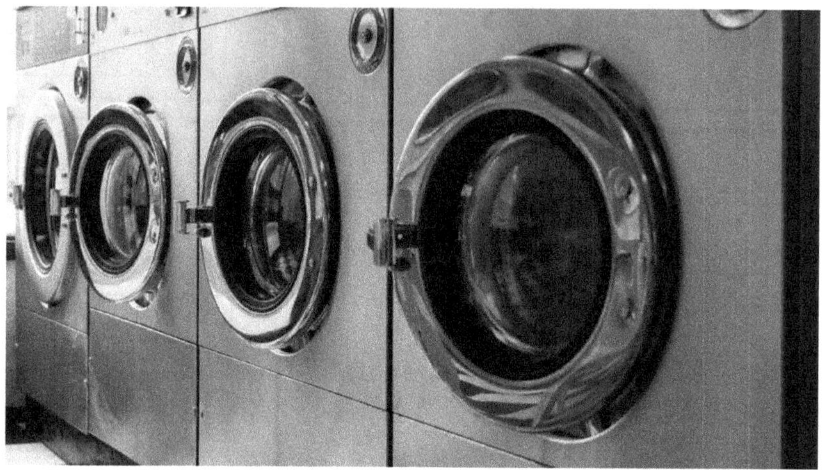

If this is a problem, you will know it because you will break out in painful hives for no reason and be referred to a dermatologist.

The laundry detergent that I am allergic to is Tide[19]. Unfortunately for me this is also the detergent used by many hotels and clothing manufacturers. I switched to

---

[19]   Tide is a trademark of Procter & Gamble

"All – Free and Clear"[20] many years ago without problems. Any "free and clear"[21] liquid detergent should be good. I also call hotels in advance and advise them of my allergy. I request they rewash the linens and towels in plain water and to not rewash them during the week. To date, they have never refused.

Less often, people sometimes find red angry streaks down their back and/or front, starting at the neck. If this happens, try a different shampoo or discontinue for a week.

---

[20] "All Free and Clear" is a trademark of Henkel Corporation

[21] Be careful that it only says, "free and clear" and not plus or anything else which will be an indicator that it may not be hypoallergenic.

<u>Foods Kill</u>

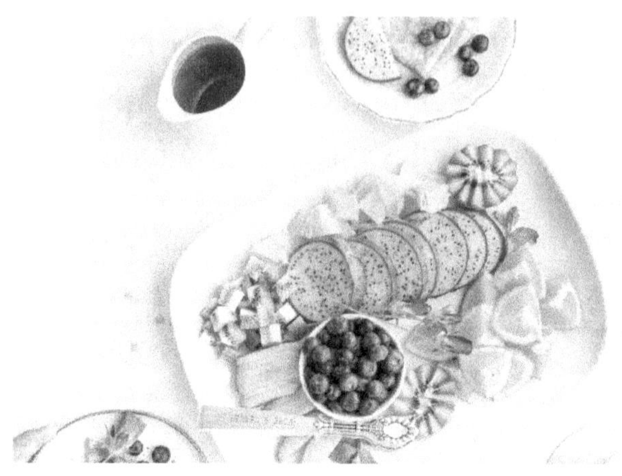

Next in line to destroy your microbiome and your health is our foods. Even unprocessed foods now contain man made poisons that directly attack the microbiome. I will get to processed foods later, for now let's discuss grains. Wheat, rye, corn, rice and many others are all grains. They are all grasses, grow vertically, they are genetically modified, they require large amounts of chemical fertilizer and they are all starchy foods. Prior to the 1970's there was nothing practically wrong with these foods and they were eaten in moderation. Now they are eaten in large quantities and they are bad for you. Eating large quantities of starch or sugar is very bad for you but eating American grains is especially bad for you. It is not just the grains from the United States but Canada, the United Kingdom, Australia and many other counties are all poisoned even before they are harvested. There are a few western countries that are holdouts, but they are under attack. The best and safest grains in the western world are from France, Italy[22] and Poland. That may change. In addition, grains from most third world countries are safe but are generally not exported.

What makes these grains so dangerous? In one word, glyphosate. Also known as Round Up ®, a chemical made by Monsanto Corporation.[23] When Monsanto created glyphosate, they didn't think it was dangerous. They bragged that you could drink it and not die. They were sort of correct, you would not die right away. Glyphosate is a weed killer. It does not directly kill weeds, but it kills the microbiome of the weeds. Without their microbiome the weeds die. Grasses like wheat would normally be considered weeds from any chemical viewpoint. That is why they were genetically modified to

---

[22] There are lawsuits in Italy to allow glyphosate, but the Italians are very fastidious about their wheat. Falsifying wheat in Italy is a crime.

[23] It appears that Bayer is purchasing Monsanto and plans to drop the name Monsanto. New name, same old problems.

resist glyphosate. In small quantities applied throughout the growing season glyphosate kills the weeds but does not kill the wheat. The wheat may absorb some of the glyphosate.

At the end of the growing season the farmer is paid more for dry wheat than for wet wheat. Significantly more since there are a lot of problems with wet wheat, deadly mold being one of them, flow in machinery being another and storage of wet wheat tends to cause fermentation and explosions. Traditionally, the farmer would just allow the wheat to naturally die and dry out or harvest it, thresh it and then dry the kernels for storage. Wheat farmers claim that in the United States about 5% of wheat crops[24] are sprayed with a dose of glyphosate large enough to kill the wheat plants which allows them to dry standing up. This is a process known as desiccating, which began in Scotland in the 1980s. Farming is a chancy business and what is normal practice at one farm or growing season may be completely different at a different farm or season. At the same time there is a large financial interest in not admitting that glyphosate is on and in our foods. Would you buy bread that you knew contained weed killer? Now the truth is that I, and many other people don't believe the 5% claim

---

[24]   https://prairiecalifornian.com/truth-toxic-wheat/

of farmers. First, they are only making that claim about desiccating and only about wheat. What about rye, corn, rice and all the other food plants? What about the glyphosate that is sprayed on the plants thought the growing season? There is a "It's a don't ask, don't tell policy' in the industry" according to Tom Ehrhardt, co-owner of Minnesota-based Albert Lea Seeds.[25] If you want to know more, I suggest you read The Organic and Non-GMO Report. (http://non-gmoreport.com)

Farmers claim that so little glyphosate is used that it shouldn't bother anyone. That may have been true at one time but not now. Glyphosate use by U.S. farmers rose from 12.5 million pounds in 1995 to 250 million pounds in 2014, a 20-fold increase. Globally, total use rose from 112.6 million pounds in 1995 to 1.65 billion in 2014, a nearly 15-fold jump.[26]

Why do I think that glyphosate survives the harvesting process to enter our bodies? I think so because the Journal of the American Medical Association (JAMA) said so. They reported levels of

---

[25] http://non-gmoreport.com/articles/grim-reaper-many-food-crops-sprayed-with-weed-killer-before-harvest/

[26] https://www.ewg.org/release/study-monsanto-s-glyphosate-most-heavily-used-weed-killer-history

glyphosate markedly increased in the bodies of a sample population over two decades. I think so because the European Union Execute Commission is concerned about it. I think so because California listed glyphosate as carcinogenic, and the World Health Organization International Agency for Research on Cancer called it "probably carcinogenic" in 2015.[27]

Let me recap how glyphosate kills weeds. It kills the microbiome of the plant which then kills the plant. What do you think glyphosate does to you when you eat it?

In addition to the food we eat that has been treated with glyphosate we eat animal products (meat, dairy, etc.) that were fed plants that were treated with glyphosate.

I could talk myself dry about glyphosate but there is no need. Glyphosate is legal, it's in almost everything we eat either directly or indirectly and you can't always prove that organic food is organic food. Organic food fraud is big business. So big that the USDA is getting involved.[28]

---

[27] https://medicalxpress.com/news/2017-10-human-glyphosate.html

[28] https://www.foodandwine.com/news/organic-food-usda-tracking-plan

<u>Preservatives</u>

Traditional Preservatives

Next let's talk about preservatives. There are traditional preservatives. These are pasteurization, dehydration, smoking, Root Cellars (refrigeration), fermentation (pickled vegetables and meats) and sea salt. Notice that none of these are poisons to bacteria. Rather they prevent bacteria from growing by providing an environment that is not suitable to them. In fact, fermentation as in pickled vegetables and traditionally dry processed fermented meats work by causing an overgrowth of beneficial bacterial and fungus which crowd out undesirable bacteria. When we eat live pickled foods, we help to replenish the beneficial bacterial that we want. Bacteria does not grow in dry desiccated foods, so dehydration and smoking create nonpoisonous environment that preserves the food. Refrigeration slows down the rate that bacteria can grow since they prefer warmth. None of these are harmful to us or our microbiome.

Gamma Radiation as a Preservative

Now let's talk about non-traditional preservatives. There are only two kinds. Irradiation and chemical. Irradiation takes several forms. One of the most common is to expose packaged foods to high level gamma radiation or x-rays or electron beams. These forms of radiation directly kill all living cells in the food without leaving any residue. The food does not become radioactive.[29] Within the United States the FDA has approved food preservation by radiation for the following[30]:

Beef and Pork

Crustaceans (e.g., lobster, shrimp, and crab)

Fresh Fruits and Vegetables

Lettuce and Spinach

Poultry

Seeds for Sprouting (e.g., for alfalfa sprouts)

Shell Eggs

---

[29] This is true in a legal sense, but food can pick up radiation, the half-life is much shorter than actual radioactive materials.

[30] https://www.fda.gov/food/resourcesforyou/consumers/ucm261680.htm

Shellfish - Molluscan

(e.g., oysters, clams, mussels, and scallops)

Spices and Seasonings

There are benefits to irradiation in that it kills the most common form of bacteria that causes food poisoning. It can be used to kill seeds (potatoes) so they don't sprout in storage. Irradiated food does not seem to bother the microbiome. Unfortunately, there is no free lunch. Irradiation works by denaturing proteins (DNA) in living cells rendering them unable to live. Some of the other chemicals normally found in living cells can be modified by the high energy radiation.[31] These products are:

- Furan, which has been linked to liver toxicity and cancer.
- 2-alkylcyclobutanones (2-ACBs), which may promote tumor growth and colon cancer; they are only in irradiated foods.

Other than the fact that irradiated food can slowly kill you the US Food and Drug Administration says it is completely safe.

---

[31] https://articles.mercola.com/sites/articles/archive/2011/11/05/why-are-your-spices--seasonings-exposed-to-half-a-billion-chest-xrays-worth-of-radiation.aspx

There is another form of irradiation, but it tends to be used mostly to purify water. That method is ultra violet radiation. It is not as high powered as the other forms and affects surface areas which works great on transparent water but not as well on solid foods which is why it may not be used as much on food. You may be most familiar with ultra violet as being a component of sunlight.

<u>Chemical Preservatives</u>

Now that we have covered radiation as a preservative it's time to cover chemical preservatives. Chemical preservatives work by killing bacteria. Your microbiome is bacteria.

I will start with one of the most common food preservatives used in cured meats, sodium nitrate[32]. This chemical kills off bacteria and changes the color of pork to pink. It is why pork lunchmeat is pink instead of grey[33]. Sodium Nitrate is naturally found in some vegetables such as spinach, radishes and lettuce. It is generally not considered dangerous unless you are intaking large amounts, are very young, have a

---

[32] Sodium Nitrite turns into Sodium Nitrate in the body, so I use these interchangeably.

[33] The natural color of all unprocessed but well drained red meats is grey. Any meat that is not grey had something added which is coloring it. A common colorant in pre-industrial processed meats are spices such as red pepper, turmeric, etc.

damaged microbiome or are taking proton pump inhibitors for acid indigestion.[34]

Sodium Nitrate[35] is poisonous if eaten in large quantities. This is very unlikely to happen. If you take a proton pump inhibitor[36] for acid ingestion or acid reflux, then this may allow for the growth of bacteria that produce nitrosamines. Nitrosamines are known to cause cancer.

Some processed meat manufacturers add ascorbic acid (vitamin C) to their products, which promotes the formation of beneficial nitric oxide instead of nitrosamines. One rather important exception is that bacon is a potential risk. Bacon contains very high amounts of nitrite and forms nitrosamines when fried at high temperatures. For this reason, only cook bacon low and slow or just don't eat it. Nitrate free bacon is also available, but it does taste a little different.

---

[34] A common proton pump inhibitor is Omeprazole, the brand name version is called Prilosec®

[35] You may have heard of sodium nitrate as being the main component of truck bombs also called fertilizer bombs. By itself, it is not combustible or explosive.

[36] Examples: omeprazole, yosprala, iansoprazole, dexlansoprazole, rabeprazole, pantoprazole.

Nitrites in large quantities can cause a condition called methemoglobinemia. Due to infant's low body weight it is hard to judge what is a large quantity and this problem mostly affects infants. The condition occurs when nitrite in the blood deactivates hemoglobin, which causes suffocation. Nitrate contamination of drinking water from nitrate fertilizer runoff is a frequent cause.[37]

Mostly nitrites are safe except in bacon or in large quantities, or if using proton pump inhibitors, or if you are an infant or your drinking water is contaminated. The U.S. Environmental Protection Agency reports that exposure to high levels of sodium nitrate has been linked to increased incidences of cancer in adults, may be related to brain tumors, leukemia and nose and throat tumors in some children. Who are you going to believe the FDA or the EPA? Both agencies end in A.

What is silly here is that the use of nitrites is totally unnecessary. All the lunchmeats that we love that use nitrites were invented in preindustrial times before nitrites were in use. In Italy, France and Germany many

---

[37] https://www.livescience.com/36057-truth-nitrites-lunch-meat-preservatives.html

meats are still process in these time-honored ways.[38] One factory in Italy traces its origin to the Roman Empire. You cannot expect imported meats to be free of nitrites since the US government regulates this.

Here is a list of the other most commonly used preservatives and their value/problems:[39]

---

[38] https://www.seriouseats.com/2016/03/salumi-guide-italian-cured-meats-salami-prosciutto.html

[39] https://www.livestrong.com/article/288335-the-most-common-food-preservatives/

BHT and BHA

Butylated hydroxyanisole (BHA) and butylated hydroxytoluene (BHT) are added to packaged foods to preserve their shelf life. BHA is used to keep high fat foods from going rancid. Examples of foods that contain BHA are butter, meat, baked goods, cereals, snack foods, dehydrated potatoes, beer and chewing gum.

Butylated hydroxytoluene (BHT) preserves foods from changing flavor, color or developing an odor. Examples of foods containing BHT are cereals, shortenings and foods high in fat and oils.

Although inconclusive so far, large doses of BHA and BHT have been shown to promote the growth of tumors in lab animals.

Sulfites

Sulfites have been used during wine making for centuries, and they are used as an antimicrobial agent and to prevent discoloration and browning in food products. Possible sources of sulfites include beer, cocktail mixes, processed baked goods, pickles, olives, salad dressing, processed salads, powdered sugar, lobster, shrimp scallops, canned clams, fruit fillings, fruit juices and potatoes. Approximately 1 in 100 individuals have adverse reactions to the preservative.

Sodium Benzoate

Sodium benzoate inhibits the growth of bacteria, mold and yeast in acidic conditions. Foods commonly using Sodium Benzoate are carbonated beverages, fruit juices, pickles, salsa and dip. Sodium Benzoate is considered safe if used in small quantities.

While the Food and Drug Administration considers these preservatives, safe there are known side effects. Preservatives protect us from food poisoning and increases the shelf life of foods which decreases their costs but some of the side effects are that they may be harmful. Bromates are known to destroy nutrients and cause diarrhea. Sulfites are known to cause joint pain and heart palpitations. Butylated hydroxytoluene (BHT) is known to cause cancer in rats. Sodium nitrate is said to cause stomach cancer, and artificially produced citric acid is said to cause asthma and allergic reactions.

In addition to these side effects the primary purpose of preservatives is to kill bacteria. Your microbiome is bacteria.

One problem with chemical preservatives is that some people only eat processed foods each of which contains preservatives. When your diet is that restricted mostly to processed foods and all of it contains preservatives then you may be eating a lot of preservatives during a day.

There is no social economic relationship between the consumption of junk/processed foods and income in the United States with some exceptions in that less educated, younger and some lower income peoples prefer processed foods. Wealthy people are as likely as poorer people to eat junk food and in general Americans eat way too much processed foods.[40]

Now we move from poisons to your microbiome to fertilizer for the bad bacterial in you that causes illness and that competes for space with your microbiome.

---

[40] https://www.ncbi.nlm.nih.gov/pmc/articles/PMC5855172/

<u>Table Sugar and High Fructose Corn Syrup</u>

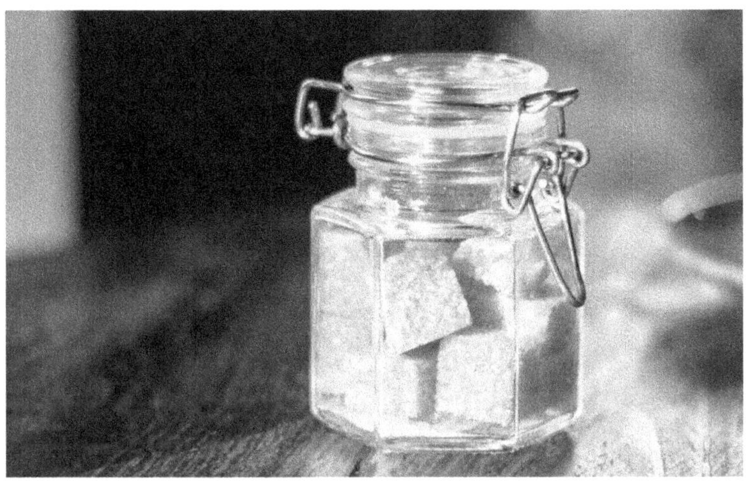

Pages 66 to 72 in my book "Dietary Fiber, essential to the human microbiome and health" I discuss sugars. Normal table sugar is called Sucrose. Sucrose is a 50/50 mix of glucose and fructose. Glucose is a sugar that your body understands and wants. When you don't have enough glucose, your body makes it from fat. Glucose is an energy source for your brain, so it is important. Fructose is the sugar that is contained in most fruits and vegetables. When eaten whole as part of the fruit it is not very dangerous in that the dietary fiber protects you from most of its effects.[41] When eaten in its

---

[41]   Therefore, I will not juice fruits.

refined form it is addictive and somewhat poisonous. Now the FDA would not call it poisonous, but I do because of its effects on the human body.

What is worse than table sugar with its 50% load of fructose is High Fructose Syrup and High Fructose Corn Syrup. These are almost all fructose. Both HFCS and HFS are banned in Europe for economic reasons since it competed with the sugar beet crops grown in Europe. This bit of larceny costs European consumers but it has the unexpected benefit of protecting their health. Larceny is a common theme in the world of sugar.

There is one book and one movie on sugar that I believe you should try to read and watch. The book is called "Pure, White, and Deadly" by Dr. Yudkin. The movie is called, "That Sugar Movie" by Damon Gameau.[42] They are both well worth the effort.

What are some of the proven[43] effects of table sugar? In one experiment conducted by Dr. Yudkin on 19 young men a sugar enriched diet produced an increase in blood triglycerides in all subjects after 2 weeks. Six of

---

[42]   If you want to go on a sugar free diet buy the movie and watch it every week. It will provide you the motivation to keep going.

[43]   "Pure, White, and Deadly", page 36, 111, 112

the subjects gained about 5lbs of weight, had an increase of blood insulin and an increase stickiness of the blood platelets. All these observations reversed within 2 weeks after the removal of sugar. That is with table sugar which is only 50% fructose.

What is the effect of HFS/HFCS (fructose) on the liver? The simple answer is devesting. The body doesn't know what to do with pure fructose without the dietary fiber it is naturally bound to. It is considered a toxin and sent to the liver. The liver doesn't need it, so it breaks it down and turns it into fat which is stored in the blood stream and the tissues of the liver. This fat raises the blood triglycerides, but it also causes Alanine Aminotransferance (ALT) enzymes to increase in the blood. ALT enzymes are used to measure liver function and damage. Increased ALT is considered to indicate increased liver damage.[44]

The increasing number of fat cells caused by the storage of HFS, signals the body to stop burning sugar since it wants to burn off the fat. Unfortunately, in the presence of HFS this backfires and causes a further increase in fat cells and/or excreting fat through the

---

[44] www.webmd.com/digestive-disorders/alanine-aminotransferance-alt#1

bowels. This causes a loss of energy/stamina and can cause mood changes including 45-minute sugar highs followed by energy crashes and sugar cravings.[45]

The United States is in an epidemic of stomach troubles. This is indicated by the fact that proton pump inhibitors (PPIs) are among the most widely used drugs worldwide.[46] Some of this can be blamed on sugar. I quote from the book "Pure, White, and Deadly";

"Large amounts of sugar, however, especially if taken in concentrated form on an otherwise empty stomach, will be an irritant.[47] You can actually see the irritation happening if you put a gastroscope into somebody's stomach, which allows you to see the stomach lining. If you now get the subject to swallow a moderately strong sugar solution – the equivalent, say, of four or five lumps in a cup of coffee – you can watch the mucous membrane turn red and angry as the irritant sugar reaches it"

---

[45]   That Sugar Film by Damon Gameau

[46]   https://www.ncbi.nlm.nih.gov/pmc/articles/PMC4864131/

[47]   Think soda and other sweetened drinks.

It is believed that sugar (fructose) is responsible for the increase of children with severe liver damage due to "fatty liver disease"[48]

Those are the direct effects of sugar on the human body. What are some of the indirect effects? Sugar changes the microbiome in a negative way and sugar changes hormones.

Let's start with the effect of sugar on the microbiome. According to the Genetics Department at the University of Utah, "several studies have turned up evidence linking obesity to the microbiome:

- A diet high in fat, sugar, and simple carbs[49] is bad for the healthy gut microbes that keep us thin while it encourages the growth of unhealthy microbes that make us obese.

- Obese individuals harbor microbes that are better at extracting energy from food, as well as microbes that signal the body to store energy as fat.

---

[48] https://www.swedish.org/blog/2015/07/fatty-liver-disease-in-children-its-about-sugar-not-fat

[49] I am going to guess that the fat is irrelevant but that is how the study was performed. They did not mention fiber.

- Bacteria transplanted from overweight mice to thin mice make the thin mice gain weight."[50]

Notice what this said, sugar changed the microbiome in a way that encourages obesity and decreased health. While not stated, I do remember that the reverse experiment was done and a change in diet with a transplanted microbiome from a thin mouse causes obese mice to lose weight. Use of microbiome transplants for this use is not approved in the United States but is under study within Europe.

This may also explain a little about why we get fat. When is the only time that sugar is high and abundant in many foods? Fall, just before the starvation period of winter. The ability to extract every calorie from food may be a survival trait given as a gift from our microbiome. The simple fact is we outsmarted ourselves and turned a survival trait into a danger.

---

[50] Genetic Science Learning Center, "The Microbiome and Disease" http://learn.genetics.utah.edu/content/microbio me/disease/

How Hormones Change Due to Sugar

Sugar can have a profound effect on certain chemicals in the body, one of which is the hormone called insulin. Insulin is secreted by the pancreas in order to turn dietary substances into glucose for the brain and heart to use. Too much sugar, however, can wreak havoc on the carefully-balanced systems of the body. Here is one way in which it can affect us on a molecular level:

"When insulin spikes, typically after a meal high in sugar, this can lead to lower levels of an important protein known as sex hormone binding globulin (SHBG). SHBG binds excess estrogen and testosterone in the blood, but when it's low, these hormone levels increase. Insulin also increases the production of testosterone, which is then converted into even more estrogen by fat tissue in the belly."[51]

---

[51] https://www.womenshealthnetworkd.com/hormonal imbalance/hormonal-imbalance-caused-by-sugar.aspx

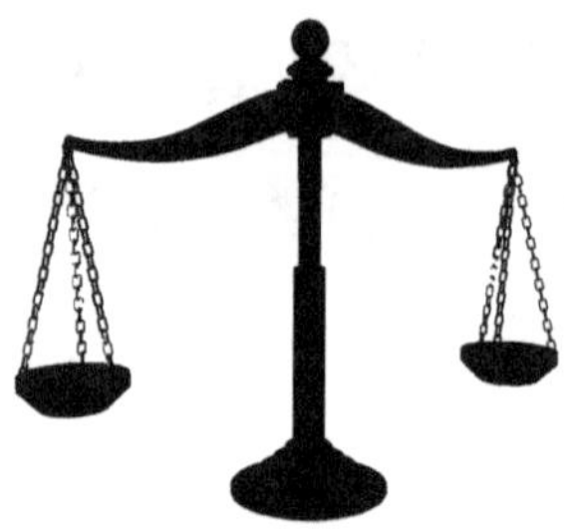

This unbalancing of the ratio of hormones in the body that affect our moods can cause us to become irritable, insomniac, and contribute to anxiety. The best thing we can do is to avoid simple sugars, like sucrose and fructose, and concentrate on eating more complex carbohydrates, fiber, protein, and good fats, which cause us to spend some energy in order to digest them in a way that simple sugars don't.

"Also, be sure to include lots of cruciferous vegetables in your diet, like Brussels sprouts, broccoli, cabbage and kale for added hormone balancing."[52]

This provides lots of fiber for your body to work on and keeps the simple sugars to a minimum.

---

[52]   https://thehealthsciencesacademy.org

<u>Identification of Sugars Hidden in Foods</u>

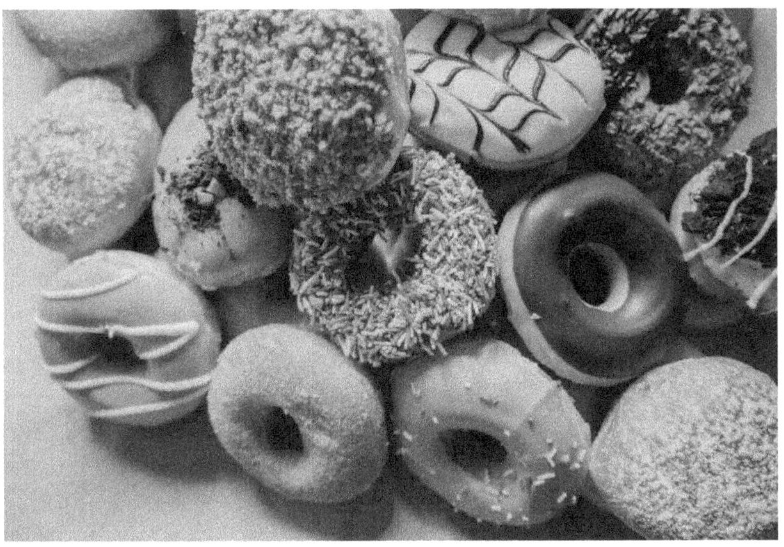

The food industry knows that people want to avoid sugar, but sugar is addictive and increases sales and therefore profits. They try to hide sugar using different names. The Health Science Academy has identified 65 alternative names used for sugar in the processed food industry. If any of these appear in the first four ingredients on a package, you know you're getting a load of sugar!

The exception to that rule is "starch", which may or may not be sugar but, in all cases, is a carbohydrate that easily converts into sugar within the body. Therefore, if you see "rich starch", "corn starch", or "potato starch", these are all simple starches that convert readily into sugars

*Agave nectar	*Dextrose	*Maltodextrin
*Agave syrup	*Diastase	*Maltotroise
*Barbados sugar	*Diastatic malt	*Maltose
*Barley malt	*Ethyl maltol	*Mannitol
*Beet sugar	*Evap. cane juice	*Maple syrup
*Brown Sugar	*Free-flowing brown sugars	*Molasses
*Buttered syrup	*Fructose	*Muscovado
*Cane crystals	*Fruit juice	*Panocha
*Cane juice	*Fruit juice conc..	*Powdered sugar
*Cane sugar	*Galactose	*Raw sugar
*Caramel	*Glucose	*Refiner's syrup
*Carob syrup	*Glucose solids	*Rice syrup
*Castor sugar	*Golden syrup	*Sorbitol
*Corn syrup	*Granulated	*Sorghum syrup

sugar

*Corn sweetener	*Grape sugar	*Starch
*Confectioner's sugar	*High fructose corn syrup	*Sucrose
*Corn syrup solids	*Honey	*Syrup
*Crystal fructose	*Icing sugar	*Table sugar
*Date sugar	*Invert sugar	*Treacle
*Dehydrated cane juice	*Lactose	*Tubinado sugar
*Demerara sugar	*Malt	*Yellow sugar
*Dextran	*Malt syrup	

<u>Artificial Sweeteners</u>

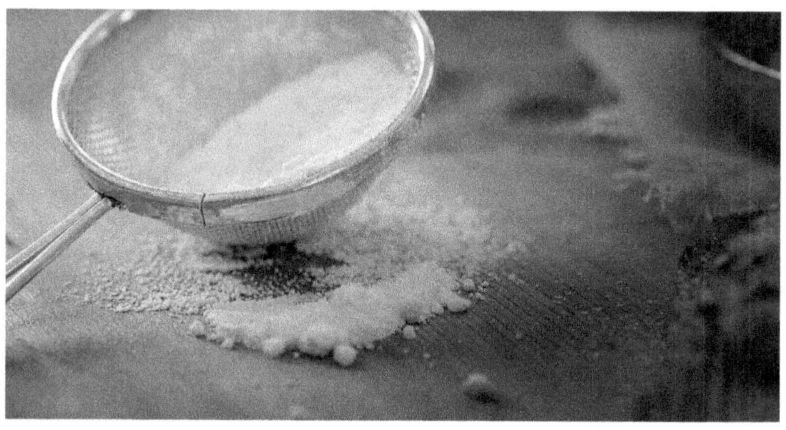

Let's talk about artificial sweeteners, I believe the safest of which is Splenda.[53]

This is counterintuitive. Everyone believes that artificial sweeteners such as Splenda are not as good for you as sugars like HFS. While they are both artificial, I believe the reserve is true that Splenda may be safer for you than High Fructose Syrup but that is not saying much. I believe that most artificial sweeteners are dangerous for many different reasons. I believe that the taste of all sweeteners triggers your body to expect the intake of high sugar foods and

---

[53] Note that I said safest, not safe. I will explain later in the chapter.

your body then reacts to that stimulus. What is the result of tricking your body into thinking you are eating high calorie sugar-based foods without the calories? Some studies indicate that since your body reacts the same it can create a sugar/insulin deficit which affects weight negatively. In other words, drinking artificially sweetened drinks might cause weight gain and still have all the bounce issues of drinking sugar laden drinks. I mentioned that I think Splenda may be safer than High Fructose Corn Syrup. **This is not an endorsement but a claim of relative safety. I equate Splenda to being shot by a gun. I equate high fructose syrup to being shot by a gun, drawn and quartered and then having your house burned to the ground with you in it.** Understand? It is a matter of relativity.

How dangerous are artificial sweeteners? There is an abundance of information available in journals and on the Internet. One of the best as far as being easy to read and understand is www.GreenMedInfo.com. They have several interesting things to say which I will paraphrase here. The Center for the Public Interest in Science downgraded Splenda from "safe" to "caution" in 2013 due to an Italian study linking the sweetener to leukemia in mice. Another peer-reviewed article titled, "Sucralose, a synthetic organochlorine sweetener: overview of biological issues" discloses an extensive list of underreported safety problem of which one of the potentially most dangerous is that Splenda when used in baking can form deadly chlorinated compounds, including dioxins. Dioxins is the well-known poison many associate with the burning of plastics. It can cause reproductive and developmental problems, damage the immune system, interfere with hormones and cause cancer. Cupcakes anyone?

So far, we have only talked about the chemical problems with Splenda but here is what I personally consider to be the scariest which I will quote from GreenMedInfo.com

"Sucralose alters indigenous bacterial balance in the Gastral Intestinal Tract": Sucralose (delivered as Splenda) has been found to reduce the number of beneficial bacteria in the gastrointestinal tract (e.g., lactobacilli, bifidobacteria), while increasing the more detrimental bacteria (e.g., enterobacteria). One study found the adverse effects on flora did not return to normal (baseline) after a 3-month recovery period. Sucralose also altered the pH of the gastrointestinal tract."

Are you kidding me? After 3 months the negative effects of Splenda on my microbiome is still not resolved? That really scares me. Does anyone even know how many months it will take for my microbiome to return to normal after drinking Splenda? Keep in mind that I think this stuff is safer than High Fructose sweeteners.

Stay away from both as much as you can. If you have a very hard time giving up HFS/HFCS and table sugar you might consider using Splenda as a transition aid.

It's Not Your Fault

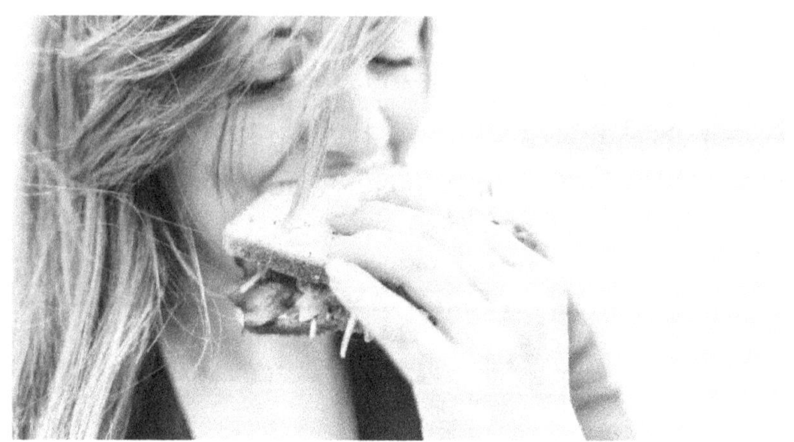

I have talked a great deal about the dangers of sugar and HFS/HFCS and how it affects the microbiome and your health. If you are old enough, you will remember that obese individuals were almost never seen in the United States prior to the 1980's. What changed, who is responsible and what can be done?

First, I want to give you a theory I have about obesity and health. People say that you become obese and that makes you unhealthy. I don't believe that theory. What I believe is that you become unhealthy, specifically your microbiome becomes unhealthy, and then you become obese as a symptom of this illness. Obesity then causes secondary illnesses. There is a lot of evidence to my theory and if it is true, then it points to a new paradigm in health care, especially in the field of obesity.

I believe that sometime in the distant future obesity will be cured with a live culture microbiome replacement along with microbiome food education. Since the future is not today, I will help you to understand microbiome food education and teach you a way to slowly transition your microbiome from unhealthy to healthy.

Who is responsible for the obesity epidemic in the United States with its consequences of heart disease, diabetes, reduced immune function and cancer? Simply, the past members of the United States Congress are responsible and caused this by a combination of greed and a lack of knowledge. A continuous series of blunders that caused a cascading effect that became what we have today. If Congress knew what the effects of their actions were, I don't believe they would have done them. It is not too late for Congress to fix this mess but instead they concentrate on patches like universal healthcare instead of providing universal health. Medical expenses could be so low that who paid became irrelevant but Congress either doesn't know or doesn't want to know. They are fixated on a railroad track leading to doom. Let me prove it.[54]

Here is how as a nation we have been destroying our microbiome and becoming obese.

1. Federal support for a low-fat diet.
2. Federal support for a high carbohydrate diet composed of grains (food pyramid).
3. Federal tariffs that made imported cane/beet sugar expensive.
4. Federal price supports that made domestic cane/beet sugar expensive.
5. Federal support for corn that made it inexpensive.
6. Very low cost of high fructose corn syrup as compared to high tariff, price supported sugar.
7. The push for low fat foods which made food bland and unappetizing forced the use of added sweeteners, specifically low priced HFCS into almost all processed foods.
8. Federal push for increased farm productivity by endorsing glyphosate, GMO foods, artificial fertilizers (nitrates). This made farming a big business requiring large capital investments.

---

[54] http://www.regina-clarke.com/10-quotes-that-explain-american-politics-by-mark-twain-others/

9. Expansion by federal and state tax authorities for inheritance taxes which made passing on of family farms untenable. Family farms tended to be traditional food growers.

10. Authorization to use anti-bacterial soaps by the Federal Government. Currently being corrected but not entirely.

11. All the above which made factory farming profitable. Factory farms meats contain very little nutrition, high concentrations of poisons and antibiotics. (low Coagulated Linoleic Acid).[55]

To back up my claims start by reading the article, "How the Ideology of Low Fat Conquered America" by Ann F. La Berge. https://academic.oup.com/jhmas/article/63/2/139/772615

Then read the book, "The Big Fat Surprise" by Nina Teicholz. Available at amazon.com and most bookstores.

President Johnson had a heart attack (November 22, 1963) most likely brought on by his 60 cigarette per day smoking habit. Blaming cigarettes was not possible back then as the cigarette lobby was powerful and rich. In addition, from around 1930 until sometime in the 1950s many American Medical Doctors not only

---

[55]   https://www.ncbi.nlm.nih.gov/pmc/articles/PMC2846864/

endorsed cigarettes but smoked themselves. This was caused by cigarette lobby fake scientific papers and endorsements. That started to end Jan. 11, 1964 with the Surgeon General's report linking smoking to certain diseases.[56] Not to allow any tragedy that captures the national interest go to waste, politicians and the federal government jumped on this to promote a heart healthy diet that supported specific high profit agriculture products over traditional products. Specifically, grains such as wheat and corn over meat and dairy.

The American Medical Association, the Diet Industry and even popular books supported the low-fat craze. This was further endorsed by the Federal Government, the food industry and popular media which pointed to flawed scientific studies. Some of these studies force fed animal fats to herbivores like rabbits. The American Heart Associate originally did not recommend a low-fat diet. They suggested substituting a substantial part of liquid vegetable oils for solid animal fats such as butter and fatty meats. At that time, corn oil was very inexpensive.

---

[56] https://www.healio.com/hematology-oncology/news/print/hemonc-today/%7B241d62a7-fe6e-4c5b-9fed-a33cc6e4bd7c%7D/cigarettes-were-once-physician-tested-approved

In 1977 the U.S. Senate's Select Committee on Nutrition and Human Needs, chaired by George McGovern, put the low-fat healthy heart theory on the national agenda with its publication of the "Dietary Goals in the United States." As McGovern stated: "Too much fat, too much sugar or salt, can be and are directly linked to heart disease, cancer, obesity and stroke." We know this to only be partly true. Too much sugar leads to heart disease by destroying the microbiome. The guide promoted increased carbohydrate and reduced fat consumption along with less sugar and salt. The report recommended that Americans eat more fruits, vegetables, whole grains, poultry, and fish, less meat, eggs, and high-fat foods, and that they substitute nonfat for whole milk. Critics, both scientific and industrial, called the diet-heart hypothesis unproved and the dietary recommendations disputable. Under pressure from many constituencies, but especially the food industry, the committee revised and reissued its report later in the year. The revision modified the cholesterol recommendations and changed the wording from the negative, such as "reduce meat consumption," to the more open, "choose meats and fish that will reduce saturated fat."[57]

---

[57] The only part of this the public seems to hear was "fat bad"

In 1917[58] the United States Department of Agriculture (USDA) laid out five basic food groups: fruits and vegetables, meats and other protein foods, cereals and other starchy foods, sweets, and fatty foods. By 1958, the food groups were reduced to four: milk, meat, vegetable/fruit, and bread/cereal. In 1941 the basic seven food groups was announced. In 1992 it introduced the Food Guide Pyramid[59] which showed carbohydrates as the suggested largest quantity of foods consumed. Why the USDA was involved in this instead of the FDA (and its predecessors) is not much of a mystery, look at the USDA charter to increase farming.[60]

You remember how dangerous sugar is? You remember how dangerous high fructose syrup is? Twice as dangerous as sugar. Why are we one of the few nations in the world to use HFS and HFCS? Congress. Congress put crazy high tariffs on imported sugar while providing high price supports for domestic

---

[58] https://www.rileychildrens.org/connections/evolution-of-usda-food-guides-to-todays-myplate

[59] To see what I consider a healthy food guide turn the USDA food pyramid upside down so what was smallest is now largest and the formally largest is now smallest.

[60] You won't be happy with the knowledge so maybe don't read it.

sugar and high subsidies for corn. The first sugar tariff was put in place in 1789 with continued support since that time. One of the latest supports was the 1990 "Farm Bill" which sets US sugar policy via price supports, preferential loans, domestic market controls and tariff quotas. The reason? The United States (U.S.) is the fifth largest sugar producer and fifth largest consumer of sugar in the world. According to the U.S. International Trade Commission, the sugar program imposes a $49 million net cost on the economy. According to a study commissioned by the Sweetener Users Association, the program costs consumers $2.9 billion to $3.5 billion. According to a study by the American Enterprise Institute, the program costs consumers $2.4 billion per year, with a net economic cost of $1 billion per year. This is big money, and everyone knows Congress loves big money. [61] [62]

High fructose corn syrup is not a naturally occurring substance. Fructose is sweeter than glucose which means it costs less than sugar on a cost basis. In

---

[61]   https://www.forbes.com/sites/timworstall/2017/01/18/if-us-sugar-tariffs-make-americans-poorer-then-donald-trumps-tariffs-will-make-americans-what/#2bd943602ec4

[62]   https://www.heritage.org/trade/report/us-trade-policy-gouges-american-sugar-consumers

addition, HFCS is cheaper than sugar because of the government farm bill corn subsidies.[63] Products with HFCS are sweeter and cheaper than products made with cane sugar. Since the turn of the millennium, Americans have paid an average of 79% more for raw sugar and 87% more for refined sugar compared to the average world price. HFCS is subsidized. Industry is not stupid. Forced to abandon fats they had to add sweetener, HFCS was much less inexpensive than sugar therefor they turned to it everywhere possible. [64]

Leaky gut, or increased intestinal permeability is not recognized by all medical doctors but there is strong scientific evidence that it is real and there are many doctors successfully treating people for it.[65] I myself was diagnosed with leaky gut and successfully treated by a medical doctor with significant health benefits.

---

[63] Your tax dollars at work making you sick

[64] https://drhyman.com/blog/2011/05/.../5-reasons-high-fructose-corn-syrup-will-kill-you/

[65] https://www.healthline.com/nutrition/is-leaky-gut-real#section6

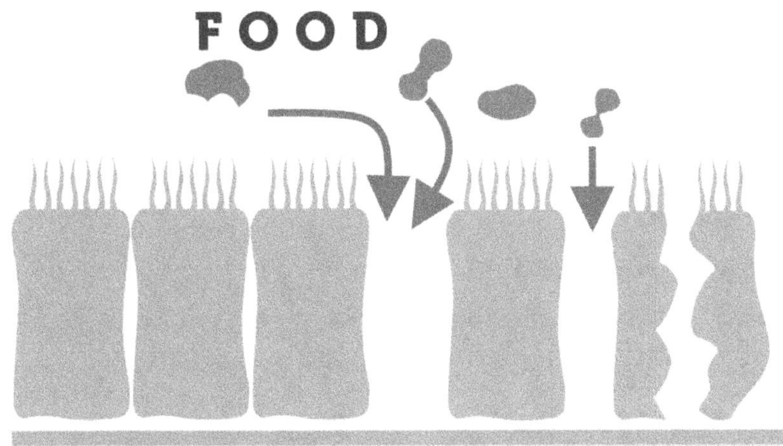

There are a lot of theories about what causes leaky gut but most of the theories center about the microbiome of the gut. Once the microbiome of the gut is damaged then the Intestinal Mucosal Cells become loose allowing molecules that would normally be too big to be absorbed into the bloodstream to enter.[66] Here are some of the things that are associated with intestinal damage to the mucosal cells: specific dietary protein, low HCL and Enzymes, antibiotic damage to microbiome, infections, blood sugar issues, overactive antibodies, pregnancy issues, menopause issues, toxins, food allergies, stress. I will explain some of these and

---

[66] https://drjockers.com/10-foods-heal-leaky-gut-syndrome/

why I believe some of them are real and some of them are false.

Specific dietary proteins like Gluten – No. I don't believe that any normal natural food proteins are the cause of leaky gut but once you have it, I do believe that many proteins that should not enter the blood steam can and the effects can be widespread including perpetuating the leaky gut by an overactive and depleted immune system with the result of low-level, even sub-clinical inflammation. Let me explain. There is a scientist that wrote a book about his discoveries that modern gluten can cause allergic reactions in the blood (where they don't belong) and that these allergic reactions can then attack the thyroid.[67] I myself was diagnosed with Hashimoto's Thyroid. The doctor I went to performed an IgE food allergy test and identified gluten as a strong allergy. He prescribed a total avoidance of gluten. I did so and four years later my thyroid function went from zero to normal. Keep in mind that was the only change. A protein was entering my blood which caused my immune system to react and suppress my thyroid. I believe that leaky gut allows molecules into the blood where they don't belong, and

---

[67] Dr. Alessio Fasano

this can masquerade as many problems including arthritis.

Low HCL and Enzymes – Maybe. This one is more difficult because low Hydrochloric Acid (HCL) in the stomach can cause live bacteria and other chemicals that are not beneficial to enter the lower digestive track where they don't belong. That can upset the microbiome. Enzymes have the same effect in that their lack can cause things to enter the lower digestive track and upset the microbiome. Do I believe that low HCL and enzymes cause an unhealthy microbiome? No, but I do believe it can contribute to it if your microbiome is already on edge. There is a possibility that low HCL and enzymes are caused by an unhealthy microbiome of the stomach lining and upper digestive track. H Pylori is a normal part of the microbiome of the stomach, however when the microbiome is damaged the H Pylori population can expand. One of the functions of H Pylori in the microbiome of the stomach is to reduce or stop acid production. It is easy to see that an overabundance of H Pylori can cause low stomach acid.[68] H Pylori is associated with stomach ulcers because the reduced acid allows bacteria that normally does not survive to attach the stomach lining.

---

[68]   https://drjockers.com/symptoms-low-stomach-acid/

Toxins – Yes. We already covered this.

Food Allergies – No and maybe. I already covered this but allow me to say that anytime there are food allergies there is inflammation and upsetment of the gut and its microbiome. This is a serious problem that feeds back into itself. The microbiome is damaged causing leaky gut which causes food allergies which cause inflammation which contributes to leaky gut.

Stress – No and maybe. At one time medical doctors believed that stress caused ulcers. That was before veterinarians taught them that it was caused by H Pylori and how to cure it. What I believe is that our gut is very sensitive to our emotions and there is a feedback loop between our emotions and the gut. The microbiome can cause and affect our emotions, so I believe that our emotions can affect our microbiome and gut. Remember the saying, "I have a gut feeling", "I feel it in my gut", "it makes my guts churn"? These old says have a truth to them. I believe that stress can cause the microbiome damage if it is already on edge or if already damaged, stress can damage it worse. At the same time, I believe that a healthy microbiome allows us to deal with stress better.

Antibiotics – Yes, but. Yes, antibiotics do damage the microbiome, but they are necessary. Modern life with antibiotics is longer, healthier and so much better. There are several problems with antibiotics:

1. Over use of antibiotics destroys the microbiome and frequent use doesn't give the microbiome time to recover. This causes a vicious feedback loop since the microbiome is about half of your immune system. A damaged microbiome can be a cause for frequent infections which require frequent antibiotics which damage the microbiome.

2. Overuse of antibiotics in our food supply can pass the effects of antibiotics on to us within meat and dairy. Not only that but the animals raised on antibiotics are not as healthy as animals that can live traditional, natural lives in pasture. This use is inexcusable and in addition it is depleting our reserves of antibiotics that work on humans by breeding super-bugs in our factory farms that become immune to antibiotics. These super-bugs then may infect us.

3. Antibiotics are known to cause weight gain. We now know this is because they damage the microbiome. In fact, this is one of the reasons that antibiotics are fed to factory farmed animals

that are not sick. The more they weight the more the corporation that owns the factory farm makes.

So, antibiotics cause damage to the microbiome with a lot of undesirable effects, but antibiotics are necessary for our health. There are many things that we can do to help us preserve our microbiome against damage. The first is to only eat antibiotic free meats and dairy. The second is to use antibiotics wisely. Some doctors will prescribe antibiotics to patients with virus infections because the patient wants the doctor to do something. Antibiotics do not work on viruses and a common viral infection does not warrant dangerous antiviral drugs. What the doctor does is issue antibiotics in order to insure no secondary infections take place. This is a waste and may prolong the virus since your immune system will eventually kill the virus. There is an old saying which is to kill a virus it takes 2 weeks without antibiotics or 14 days with.

Here is another warning. Elderly people need to take special care of their microbiome. I have seen cases where an elderly person caught an infection which was treated but because the base cause of the infection was not resolved it became a routine issue with treatment and spiraling decrease in health resulting eventually in death. This is especially true with Urinary Tract Infections which seem to become more common in the elderly. Please seek a competent medical urologist. If they don't solve the problem, switch practices to a different city and get a second opinion.

The microbiome not only has significant influence over your immune system, hormonal system, digestive system but it helps to control the way you think. This is especially true when what you are thinking about is food but there is evidence that it can affect physical age, sleep patterns and circadian rhythm.[69] When you are craving candy, sugary drinks or just sweets in general that is the bad bacteria in your gut telling your brain to eat more sugar. When you kill off the bad bacterial that wants sugar then sugar cravings end. Did you ever crave specific foods? Again, that is normally your gut microbiome telling your brain that something is needed. If you ever craved chocolate but not sugar, then that is your body telling you that either you need magnesium or that you are unhappy and want the chemical Phenylethylamine. If the craving goes away after taking a magnesium supplement, then you know which. Phenylethylamine is jokingly

---

[69] See page 61 of my book, "Dietary Fiber: Essential to the Human Microbiome and Health".

referred to as the love drug because it causes feeling like those of love. Phenylethylamine is in chocolate.[70]

The way the gut microbiome talks to your brain is complex. There are two pathways. The slow path is by release of signaling chemicals into the bloodstream. The fast way is by means of the Vagus nerve which makes a direct connection between the gut and the brain stem. This nerve pathway is so fast that signals travel from intestines to the brain stem in under 100 milliseconds.

Appetite disorders (obesity, bulimia), arthritis (nightshade plants) and some forms of depression are believed to start in the gut and be directly tied to the microbiome and food intake. I believe that malfunction of the microbiome can be involved in unhappiness and some emotional/mental issues. There are three steps involved in being happy. The first is a healthy microbiome. I do not believe that a healthy microbiome can make you happy, but I do believe that an unhealthy microbiome can make you unhappy, even depressed. The second thing is the realization that societies' social pressures, especially commercial marketing, preys upon

---

[70] https://www.amanochocolate.com/faqs/why-does-chocolate-make-people-happy/

unhappiness. They want you to be unhappy in order to convince you to spend money to be happy. Once you realize how artificial this pressure is, the desire to spend money for happiness goes away. The final part to being happy is to understand that happiness is internal. You must decide to be happy. Once you have internalized the decision, fake it until you make it. Try it, it works.

Now that you not only know that the microbiome is directly connect to your brain stem but exactly how and how fast that connection works, we can discuss things that can assist or inhibit that communications. It turns out that a common food chemical called glutamate is a neurotransmitter which might be involved as a messenger between the microbiome and the brain. Our food contains two forms of glutamates, synthetic and natural. They are not the same.[71] Natural glutamate can be found in foods as various forms of glutamic acid. It is commonly found in foods such as kelp, seaweeds, fish sauce, soy sauce, parmesan cheese[72], Roquefort cheese, dried shiitake mushrooms, miso, green tea, anchovies, cured ham, sardines, cheddar cheese, tomatoes, and

---

[71] https://naturallysavvy.com/eat/monosodium-glutamate-natural-vs-synthetic/

[72] Parmigiano-Reggiano can be eaten by those that are lactose-intolerant.

peas. Synthetic glutamates are almost always Monosodium Glutamate (MSG). You may know this as the additive in Chinese food that is now rarely used because of adverse reactions. The adverse reactions to excessive MSG have been seizures, brain cell death and anaphylaxis shock. Excessive glutamate is one of the primary reasons that people with strokes suffer brain damage. While too much glutamate is dangerous so is too little. Too little glutamate can cause psychosis, coma and death.[73]

The simple answer is that if you want to enhance the operation of your Vagus nerve, eat some foods that contain natural glutamates while being careful to not overdose.

---

[73] https://neuroanthropology.net/2008/02/25/glutamate-and-schizophrenia/

Peter V. Radatti

<u>How to Correct the Microbiome</u>

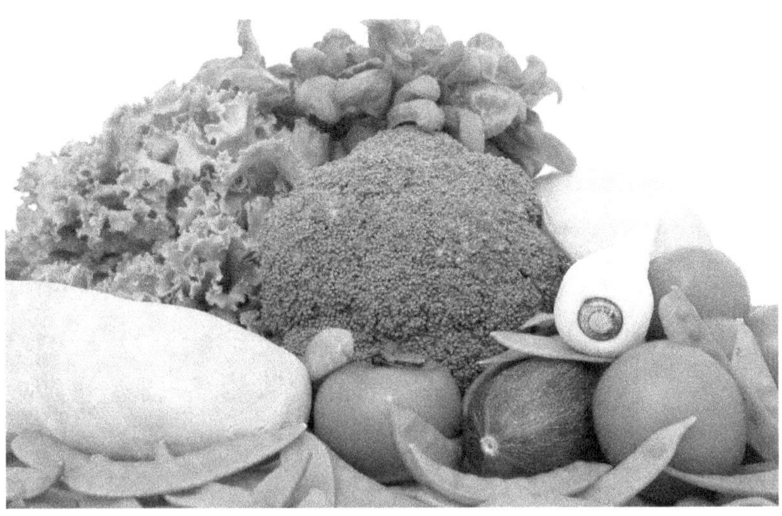

So far all I have told you about is the critical importance of your microbiome and what you do that can cause it to go wrong. This is critical knowledge because, look around. The microbiome is going wrong for a lot of people. I would be remiss if I didn't tell you what to do to protect your microbiome. First there are two words you need to know and while they sound alike, they have very different meanings. Those words are prebiotic and probiotic. The common suffix of both words is "biotic" which means referring to life. Think of the word <u>bio</u>logy. The prefix "pre" means before and the prefix "pro" means "of" or referring-to. Therefore, a prebiotic means "before life" while probiotic means "of life". Prebiotics are food for life and probiotics are alive.

The single more important thing you can do to protect and nurture your microbiome is to insure you eat a high fiber diet. Mixed dietary fiber is the food that your microbiome eats and therefor is a prebiotic. You need both water soluble and water insoluble dietary fiber. The bacteria digest dietary fiber and produces chemicals that we need as a byproduct. Dietary fiber is not digested by us therefore has no effective calories to us. Your microbiome can put up with a lot if it is well fed. Another thing you can do is to eliminate as many preservatives and glyphosate as possible. Then, stop feeding the bad bacteria in your microbiome that competes with the good bacteria by eliminating sugar as much as possible. You know you have an overgrowth of the bad bacteria if you crave sweets. When you use antibiotics be sure to supplement your microbiome with both dietary fiber (prebiotics) and with probiotics. Discuss with your doctor or pharmacist how long the antibiotic is active in your body and insure you use the probiotic longer than that time frame. A probiotic is actual live bacteria that you can add to your diet to correct a damaged microbiome. You can take a probiotic at the same time as antibiotics but if you are actively using antibiotics then taking expensive probiotics may be a little bit of a waste in that they will be rapidly killed. You will still get some benefits before they are killed off so make the cost benefit judgement yourself.

How long does it take to see results in your microbiome? You may not believe it but only 24-hours is enough for your microbiome to visibly start to correct after the addition of enough prebiotic dietary fiber. The process will then continue until you reach balance. How long before you reach balance? Unknown since environmental issues of what you eat and what you do (antibiotics, preservatives and antibiotic soaps) have an effect. The less you ingest poisons to your microbiome the faster it will reach an ideal balance. Once your microbiome reaches a certain point (which will be different for each of us) you will start to notice positive changes in your health, emotions, clarity of thought processes and the start of correction to existing problems such as obesity.

<u>Late Breaking Information</u>

This information came out too late to be added to the book, so I added this section.

GMO DNA Modification

There is enough information to write 3 or 4 more of these books with new information coming out all the time. Just as I finished this book Far Eastern Federal University (FEFU)[74] announced the results of their research on human ingestion of genetically modified foods. They found that GMO foods modified the DNA of the bacteria that comprises the microbiome in the human body. They also found that some of this modified DNA enters the blood stream with unknown results.

Micro-Plastics

A micro-plastic is any piece of plastic smaller than 5 millimeters in size. They usually get that way from

---

[74] Far Eastern Federal University is a university located in Vladivostok, Primorsky Krai, Russia. FEFU was established in 1899.

disintegration of larger pieces of plastic. Your laundry also washes a great deal of plastic lint down the drain.

There are five main types of micro-plastics: fibers, microbeads, fragments, nurdles and foam. The difference between these are mostly just shape.

According to a 2018 review entitled "Microplastics in Seafood and the Implications for Human Health"[75] about 8 million metric tons of plastic enter the oceans annually with a conservative guess that there are currently 5.25 trillion micro-plastic particles on the ocean's surfaces.

What are the dangers of micro-plastics? The same study stated that, "Following oral exposure, nano-plastics are transported by M cells, specialized epithelial cells of the mucosa, from the gut into the blood where they are carried through the lymphatic system and into the liver and gall bladder." Due to their very small size and the fact they do not dissolve in water these plastics are able to pass through the blood-brain barrier, the placenta, the gastrointestinal track and the lungs. Studies outside of the body have indicated that these particles can harm lung, liver and brain cells.

Different studies have reported toxicity in human gut, lung, liver, brain, reproductive systems including possible damage to cardiopulmonary, endogenous

---

[75] https://www.ncbi.nlm.nih.gov/pubmed/30116998

metabolites, genotoxicity (destruction of cell's DNA and RNA), inflammatory issues, oxidative stress (free radicals), nutrient absorption and damage to the microbiome.

There is no escape by eating only land-based foods. According to a report in 2017 Scientific Reports micro-plastics have been found in oceans, rivers, sediments, sewage, soil and table salt. Another study found that almost all plastic bottled water contains micro-plastics. Mice studies have proven that these plastics can accumulate in the liver, kidney and gut. They conclude that this may cause problems to energy and fat metabolism, oxidative stress and neurotoxic responses which damage nerve tissue. There are substantially more problems being discovered with health and micro-plastics but that is a subject that could take another entire book. One "good" sign is that apparently one study[76] found that some micro-plastics can be extracted in the stool. The bad news from the Environmental Agency Austria is that "more than 50% of the world population might have microplastics in their stools".

The problem of micro-plastics is far ranging and not well understood. It is a newly discovered problem, and no one knows how much of a problem it is, yet.

---

[76] Study was done by the Medical University of Vienna in Europe, Russia and Japan.

There is no avoiding micro-plastics. They are everywhere. About the only thing you can do is avoid the easy sources such as plastic water bottles, Styrofoam cups, don't cook in plastic and avoid skin products that contain "micro-beads" unless the microbeads are plant based. If you are very concerned, consider a reverse osmosis filter for your tap drinking water.

Those Pesky Parasites, What Should You Do?

by Dr. Dean Howell, ND

Dr. Dean Howell received his degree as a naturopathic physician from Bastyr University in 1982, after earning a bachelor's degree in mathematics.   Dr. Howell brought a mathematical perspective to medicine that created his quest for simplicity and empirical certainty in healing. Having taken very seriously the Hippocratic oath which included the injunction to treat the cause rather than the symptoms of the disease or condition, Dr. Howell has striven to discover more precise methodologies that lead to permanent and cumulative beneficial results. NeuroCranial Restructuring, which Dr. Howell has been developing for over 30 years, is a powerful and dynamic new approach to physical medicine with broad application. Its effectiveness continues to increase as he incorporates more cutting-edge strategies into its operation.

Dr. Howell, the developer of NeuroCranial Restructuring, is a licensed naturopathic physician. He divides his time between Los Angeles, California and Tonasket, Washington state. Visit his website for more information: http://drdeanhowell.com/

Those of you who have seen me recently know that my health has soared over the last years. Not only have I lost more than 110 pounds of weight, I have been growing more hair on my head, my gray and silver hair has been gradually turning back to the light brown/dark blonde color that I had in my 30s, the age spots on my hands have faded, I am growing new veins to replace the varicose veins in my legs, and my personality is less arrogant and more approachable than I had been in the past.

People want to know: "What have you done?"

First, let me say that it has not been easy. Do not believe anybody who tries to sell you seemingly magic pills and potions, or a simple diet that will somehow transform you into a slender, healthy person. It just isn't so! However, it is also not a process that requires tremendous self-control.

Let me give you a little background, so that you can understand my advice a little better: by the time I reached age 2, I was fighting chronic bronchitis. At age 3 they removed my tonsils.

I continued having bronchitis recurrently throughout the fall and winter every year. At age 6½ I received my second vaccine, this one for smallpox. Nobody understood why, but my weight increased 40% in the next three months! I went from 62 pounds to 96 pounds from September to January. Since that time, I have battled being fat. Perhaps you had some sort of affliction too? If so, then, you can understand how uncomfortable and painful it could be for a boy who is teased about being fat. The only way that I could lose weight was to starve.

I last took antibiotics when I was 17. I decided to starve myself skinny, and I lost a lot of weight I found out that I was "fasting." For me, fasting meant having almost continuous cramping in my lower abdomen, and waking up with bruised teeth and gums from the grinding and clenching that I would go through all night. When I went to medical school, my instructors assured me that this was an emotional reaction to the lack of food and that I should not worry, so I didn't worry about it.

Many medical students believe that they have many of the diseases that they study in pathology class. I did that, too. When I studied about yeast, fungi, and parasites, I became convinced that I had them. I had one of my clinical laboratory instructors who proclaimed himself an expert in parasite detection (because of his experience running a parasitic disease unit for the Royal Canadian Navy during World War I). He pronounced me parasite-free but said that I was loaded with fungi. "Fortunately," he said, "You have no Candida. The kind of fungi living in you is a tree-loving fungus that is not pathogenic for humans."

My other teacher in medical laboratory diagnosis taught me that the total amount of fungus in my poop should be between 5-10% of the total volume of the biome (the mucus lining of the intestinal tract where bacteria, fungus, yeast, and parasites live).

Both teachers assured me that I was okay, and this fungus was not a problem. I continued living as I had lived since I was 20 years old, eating a diet of 30% fat, 30% protein, and 40% carbohydrates.

I love to read. My favorite reading tends to be fiction that is placed in the historical, real world. I read a book series about "The Clan of the Cave Bear." I found the writing about humans living 30,000 years ago so fascinating that I ended up reading more of the scientific background that the author also read.

Humans have lived on the earth for several million years, living as hunter-gatherers. For the most part, this meant that we lived in three or four locations per year, moving from place to place, often moving with the seasons. We moved in this fashion because of the food that would be available at each location, visiting each location when the foods there was ripe. Winters we lived in caves and underground dwellings to protect us from animals and the severe cold that we often had with the ice ages. For example, humans lived in limestone caves in central France. But they only lived in their caves during the wintertime, living in other locations the rest of the year. As the humans moved from place to place, they ate the fresh food that was in season, and then preserved food by dehydration and smoking, taking this with them to survive the winter. During the ice ages, there was permafrost below the ground that would serve like a refrigerator for fresh meats. For the most part, we would dehydrate (dry) fresh meats, fruits, and even vegetables to eat during the long, cold winter.

But what these "primitive" people could not do was to farm. To farm required them to stay in one place the entire year, and they could not sustain their whole tribe without traveling. After all, once you killed all the animals in the woods around your camp, what would you eat after that? At one time, there was species of cattle called aurochs that averaged over 1 ton each. Sometimes the tip of their horns were 7 feet across!

Years ago, all the aurochs were apparently killed. I guess there were no environmentalists to stop the complete decimation of the aurochs.

During these many, many years, people did not die from heart disease, cancer, nor diabetes, nor neurologic diseases. Instead, they would die of other, more natural conditions, such as starvation, infections, animalattacks, human attacks and so forth. Consider their diet: they primarily ate dried meats, some dried fruits, some dried vegetables, and, perhaps, some roots like yams and potatoes that they may have found. But, because they were so often on the move, there was no way for them to farm. After all, animals will ravage the farm if you are not there to protect it and these people moved 3 to 5 times per year. So as recently as 30,000 years ago, humans lived without animals. This means that they were in the early stages of beginning to work with dogs, horses, chickens, ducks, geese, cattle, goats, sheep, and other animals which were all only seen in the wild, and were occasionally killed and eaten, their body parts used for meat, tools, clothing, and furniture.

I suspect that their diets were rarely more than 10% carbohydrate (but the scientists that I have read failed to speculate about this). Others have written about this, and the paleolithic diets were created from their writings. This means that they rarely needed to secrete insulin. Insulin is the hormone that we secrete to prevent our blood sugar from going too high and damaging us. Insulin causes inflammation. It was probably only during the seasonal festivals that anybody worked hard enough to gather enough grass seeds or grapes to make beer or wine. Since they did not farm, finding roots like yams, turnips, pursed lips, or potatoes was not a regular occurrence. According to the scientists, they were not eating grains, they were making them into beer.

So, it was probably the desire of men to drink beer that caused them to develop a farming way of life, allowing them to protect their fields from ravaging deer and cattle so that they could make beer, and even eat the grains! THIS BEGAN HAPPENING ONLY 10 to 12,000 years ago!

Since humans have lived on Earth for millions of years, our biochemistry is still that of a hunter and gatherer, because 12,000 years is a very short time compared to millions of years.

When I was in medical school, I was told that I must eat a diet composed of carbohydrates, fats, and proteins, and that eating too much protein would be damaging to my body. Even more, they taught that a simple diet of primarily meat would leave us with severe nutritional deficiencies that could only be solved through the consumption of the appropriate vegetables and herbs. Looking at the history that I told you just above, where did these experts come up with these peculiar ideas? They claimed that these were scientifically validated, but now I was beginning to wonder if that was true.

I began reading more widely. There was a famous physician who brought homeopathy from Germany to the United States in the 1840s. His name was Constantin Hering. He wrote that parasitic infections were universal – that all his patients had them, and that he had seen them in their dead bodies as well. He decided whether to treat patients for parasites based on his examination of their poop. He wrote that if there were only two or three visible worms in their poop, then it was not bad enough to treat.

Over the past 40 years, then, I tried many methods to kill off the excessive fungi in my colon. I tried herbs, I tried medications, I tried homeopathic medicines, I tried energy treatments, I tried electrical treatments, I tried radio wave treatments, all without results. There was always a craving in the bottom of my abdomen. Something was calling to me, "It's time to eat simple carbohydrates!" After I had eaten a large Thanksgiving dinner, somehow there was still room for dessert. When I denied myself access to sugar, I would binge on fruits. One of my favorite breakfasts 35 years ago was to cut up grapes, papayas, bananas, mangoes, apples, pears, raisins, dates, nuts, and then cover the fruit with dried chipped coconut, and then coat it all heavily in plain yogurt. In those days, I believed that that was a healthy meal!

Ten years ago, my second wife was diagnosed with cancer and my life went to hell. She tried a blend of mainstream medicine and alternative medicine and it went very badly. When her weight got very low, she asked me to cook her favorite meals for her, and then would still not eat very much. Because of my emotional state, and my inability to waste food, I ended up eating more and more. After she died, I got even fatter by eating at least five pints of Häagen-Dazs ice cream every week. One night I woke up at 3 AM standing in front of the open refrigerator with its bright light shining in my eyes, with food in both hands and my mouth full of food. I was sleep eating! It happened a few more times in the following week. I started thinking that I was going to have to chain myself to the bed or put a padlock on the refrigerator.

Then I began thinking about parasites, bad bacteria, and the amount of fungus that was living in my digestive tract – maybe that was the problem! When I tried to selectively kill off bacteria or fungi, I met with no success. When I thought about the bacteria that were probably living in my digestive tract, I realized that those bacteria were the survivors of all the antibiotics that I took 2 to 3 times a year in my youth. I had taken no antibiotics since age 17. And here I was, nearly 60 years old, with a horrible biome.

I wondered why it was important to save these bacteria. Couldn't I replace them with something better? When I had tried probiotics, I noticed no change, but my poop was sure expensive! Instead, I decided to kill everything in my digestive tract.

I called it "Taking the Nuclear Option." I decided to get an ozone machine and to perform a technique called rectal insufflation. This meant that I got 1-1/2 quarts of very clean water that was very warm and put it into my enema bucket. Then I had a traditional enema. Afterwards, I sat on the toilet until the dirty water ran out. Then I used a male urinary catheter, (which is made from silicone) and attached it to the end of the outflow of ozone hose from the ozone machine. I sent the ozone regulator to a flow rate of 0.5 liters per minute. Then I inserted the urinary catheter into my rectum and laid on my right side on the floor. Once in place I turned on the ozone machine and tried to get in at least 1 liter of the ozone gas. This takes two minutes. Sometimes I wouldn't get in quite that much, and a few times I was able to put in more. I tried to hold still after turning off the ozone machine and if I lasted two or more minutes before needing to release the gas from my colon, then the gas smelled like air and did not smell like ozone.

One day I had a lot of pain after I had administered the ozone. This was unusual. A while later, I noticed that I needed to poop again. This was also unusual. I sat on the toilet and strained and out came a worm! It was almost as long and thick as a pencil, and it had a top that resembled a palm tree. That was the only day that anything came out after administering the ozone.

At first, I would get a blinding headache for 2 to 4 hours after every ozone insufflation. After 100 (or so) treatments, I was feeling much better, and had no reaction at all from doing the ozone therapy. I noticed that I did not crave carbohydrates. I did not have to eat late at night, nor did I wake up sleep eating. I did not crave ice cream.

But I was afraid to stop, so I did this for a few more months whenever I was home. Finally, I decided it was time, and I ate a lot of probiotic pills, plain grass-fed yogurt, plain grass-fed kefir, some fermented foods, and even had enemas of probiotics. During the next year, every month I would feel a little better than I had the month before. I was much better for two years after this.

Last winter I noticed that Häagen-Dazs was more attractive to me when I would walk past it the grocery store. This was alarming since each ozone treatment took me at least an hour, I was not anxious to resume that much work. When I went to my Brooklyn office to work, and my assistant there, Rebecca Hart-Malter was bouncing around her shop as I had never seen her behave before. She was so excited, and she had so much more energy than I had come to expect from her. She told me that her guides (she is a medical intuitive and psychic) told her to investigate turpentine and kerosene. When she researched them online, she found out that they had been used for many years to kill yeast, fungi, bacteria, and parasites. She showed me Ziploc bags with the roundworms that she had pulled out of the toilet after she had pooped. I realized that I had a quicker option to kill my new, bad biome.

After I left Brooklyn, I went to Denver to work at my next stop in Boulder, and then went to Home Depot and purchased commercial turpentine. When there, I discovered that there were two cans right next to each other and one was labeled turpentine, which had distilled pine oil with methylene and xylene added, and turpentine, which was 100% pure distilled pine oil. Since I knew that methylene and xylene are deadly poisons, I bought turpentine. The articles that we read online did not always agree with each other, but it appeared the consensus was that the appropriate oral dosage was 1-3 tablespoons of turpentine daily. Many people work up gradually because they feel flu-like and/or have headaches if they took too much too soon.

Since I had a history of having killed yeast, fungus, parasites, and bacteria, I decided that I could start it up and take that dosage quite soon. I took 2 tablespoons the first day, and the next morning I had a diarrhea movement that had a 10- inch worm which looked like a fern leaf floating on the surface of the diarrhea. My craving for ice cream was already gone! I continued to take 2 tablespoons of turpentine once daily, finding that it was best to take it on an empty stomach, if I was hungry, I could eat a couple hours later without any problem. I did this until the next full moon, which took almost a month.

Have you ever heard the police say that the time of the full moon is when there are the most violent crimes? It may be because of increased parasite activity. Parasites change our behavior by secreting chemicals into our bloodstreams. Another interesting characteristic of worms and other parasites is that the adults may lay many eggs, depending on the quality of their diet – which is best with a lot of simple carbohydrates. The more simple-carbohydrates that you consume, the more eggs are laid and, especially when you kill the parents, new eggs will hatch around the days near the date of the full moon. As far as I have been able to discover, yeast, fungus, and bacteria are not so predictable.

Once again, it was time to build a new biome. I now realized that the choice of probiotics was crucial for the development of the new biome. Essentially, killing everything in your digestive tract is like preparing soil for a new garden. There are no seeds in the dirt, until you choose them. This time I selected multiple strains of bacteria that I considered good choices and took lots of them the first few days after stopping the turpentine. I tried to take more probiotics every hour or two. It was rather like continually sprinkling more seeds over the garden. You don't want too many in each place, but you want to make sure that they are well installed in your soil. Then, your diet provides the nutrients and fertilization for the new bacterial biome. Unlike worms, who only eat from your lymphatics and blood stream, the bacteria eat from food residues.

There are authors out there who will maintain that consuming sugar along with the turpentine will kill parasites more effectively. This is nonsense, because the parasites have no mouths to eat the sugar, meat, or other residues from your diet, substances like sugar are absorbed into the bloodstream quickly from the stomach. The parasites don't notice a teaspoon or so of sugar in your diet, because a teaspoon of sugar is not enough to raise your blood glucose levels. If you wish to consume more dessert, or a whole quart of Pepsi, the parasites and fungus sent signals through your bloodstream to change your brain function so that you will eat lots of these carbohydrates. In this way they can have sex and party! This allows the parasites to lay more eggs, which makes sure that they can live in you for a long time!

There are also authors who will maintain that parasites are beneficial. Again, this is nonsense. We have three relationships with other animals: symbiotic (where both parties receive benefits, like the good bacteria in our biome), commensal (where we live together and neither party affects the other), and parasitic (where the parasite takes from the host and the host receives no benefit). Parasites are, by definition, very bad.

This time, with superior choice of probiotics, my hair color changed, the size of my bald spot lessened, the veins in my legs healed more, the age spot in my hands faded. Rebecca noted that she felt mentally clear when we chose the right probiotics for her.

Rebecca and I are noticing huge improvements with these parasite and biome rebuilding protocols. Not just for us, but for many people who tried this in order to recover from diseases.

---End Chapter---

LEGAL NOTICE: Do not attempt to use turpentine or any other substance without medical supervision. Doing so may result in harm and/or death. Only a licensed Doctor can advise you.

Questions From Reviewers on Taking Turpentine:

Should I follow what Dr. Howell did?

Answer: No. Dr. Howell is a licensed Naturopathic Doctor and unless you are also a licensed Doctor you do not have the skills necessary to do what he did for himself. Dr. Howell did not provide a protocol, he provided a true account of his experience and nothing more.

Should I drink Turpentine?

Answer: No. Here is one entry from the Merck's Manual of the year 1899:[77]

Oil, Turpentine, Rectified, Merck.—U.S.P.

For *internal* use only the *rectified* oil answers.—**Dose:** 5—30 ℳ; for tapeworm, 1—2 drams.—*Preparation:* Lin. (35%, with 65% resin cerate).

> Here is what the U.S. National Institute of Heath, National Library of Medicine[78] in the year 2019 says:

---

[77] https://www.gutenberg.org/files/41697/41697-h/41697-h.htm

Turpentine oil poisoning

Turpentine oil comes from a substance in pine trees. Turpentine oil poisoning occurs when someone swallows turpentine oil or breathes in the fumes. Breathing these fumes on purpose is sometimes called "huffing" or "bagging." It is a member of a class of compounds known as hydrocarbons. Exposure to hydrocarbons, both intentional and unintentional, is a common problem resulting in thousands of calls to poison control centers each year.

I see a lot of videos about Turpentine as medicine on YouTube. Should I follow these directions?

Answer: I also saw these videos and the primary person creating these videos is a Medical Doctor. I am not a medical doctor and do not have the legal right to advise you. Seek advice from a Medical Doctor.

In attempting to answer these questions I searched Google, YouTube and Amazon.Com for" Turpentine" or "Turpentine as Medicine" and got a great deal of confusing answers. I also personally met licensed Medical Doctors from other countries that ingest turpentine themselves but are careful to use herbal brands and not hardware store brands. I have found

---

[78] https://medlineplus.gov/ency/article/002746.htm

that turpentine is a common ingredient for topical ointments such as old fashion liniment (still commercially available) and also very effective for bug bite relief. While I have no idea if it is true and can only read the automated translations, there seems to be a great deal of information on the use of turpentine as medicine in the French and Russian languages. If you are determined to do this then seek medical supervision from a licensed doctor.

Finally, I believe Dr. Howell to be a man of great personal integrity and beliefs. I am certain that what he related actually happened the way he described and as attributed.

<u>Weight Loss</u>

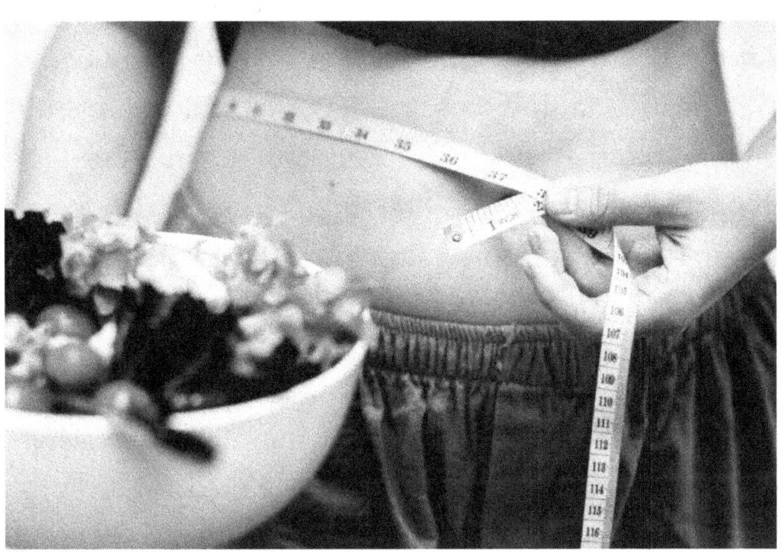

I am going to finish this book with a weight loss diet that is microbiome friendly, allows you to eat a variety of foods including fruits and vegetables all while you lose about 1 pound (approximately. 0.5 Kilograms) per day, every day, without a plateau, if you follow it. Results vary, especially if you make mistakes. This is the diet that I follow. This diet is called a modified Pescatarian Diet. I did not invent it. It is mostly low carbohydrate since you are not eating any grains or sugar, except you are allowed certain fruits. It is not vegetarian since you are eating flesh in the form of fish and seafood but no land-based protein.

You are eating dietary fiber in the form of vegetables and fruit plus there are bonuses that you can eat that increase your fiber intake. This diet is sort-of ketogenic since it is unusually low in carbohydrates and the fats are mostly natural fats in the fish which are anti-inflammatory. You are allowed some bonus fats. The diet is almost a paleo diet but both more restrictive and easier. There are some cakes and sweets that you can eat but the brands you can eat are limited.

Exercise is not necessary for this diet to work but it is strongly recommended. If nothing else, moderate exercise will help you emotionally. My preferred exercise is walking.

All weight loss diets and programs are serious business. You are modifying your body and health therefor it needs to be constantly monitored by a medical doctor. The same is true of exercise. If you are not used to exercise, talk with your doctor first. **Do not start this diet without consultation with a Medical Doctor.**

Weight loss diets <u>are not</u> a lifelong diet. If you stayed on the diet too long you will go from an unhealthy overweight to an equally unhealthy under-weight. In addition, this diet is very restrictive so please discuss with your medical doctor taking supplemental vitamins. The supplements I take are Vitamins D and B-Complex.

If you decide to take a break from this diet as I have, then stay on the Ketogenic diet. I didn't lose weight on Keto, but I didn't gain weight and I consider that a win. No one can eat the same all the time. When I lost 30 pounds, I gave myself a break for a few weeks where I ate steak, lamb and other red meats. I did not gain any weight during the break.

Once you get your weight where you want it, discuss with your doctor how to maintain it.

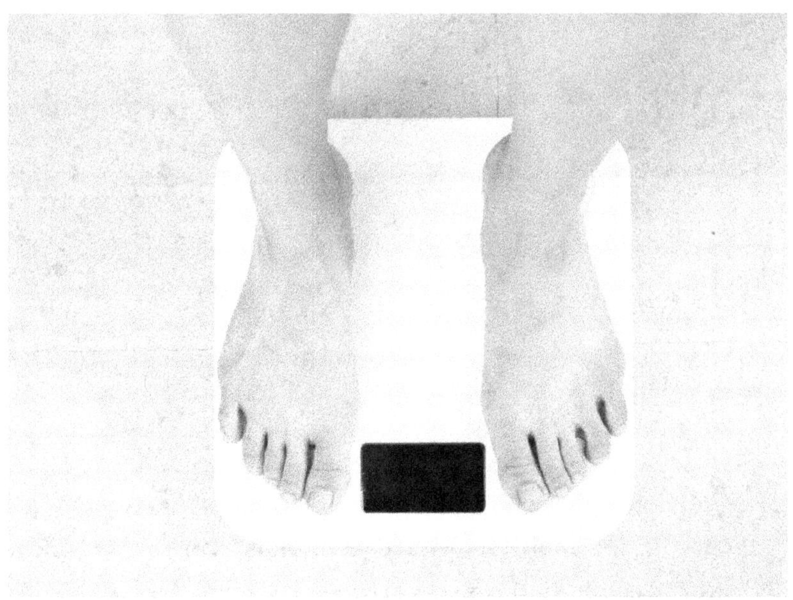

Here is the basic diet:

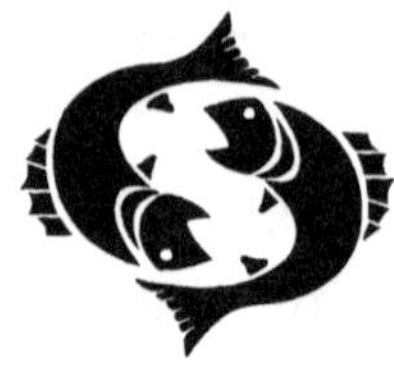

Pete's Pescatarian Weight Loss Diet

Time	**Action**
Upon Waking	Drink 1 glass of water
Sometime AM	Drink 1 cup of coffee or tea. Nondairy Coffee-mate is allowed as is flavoring. (If constipated drink coffee or additional water or consider an OTC drug)[79]
9:00 AM	Eat a fruit of the type specified
12:00 Noon	Eat seafood and vegetable of the types specified
3:00 PM	Eat a fruit of the type specified
6:00 PM	Eat seafood and vegetable of the types specified

---

[79] This is optional. If your doctor tells you to not drink coffee or tea then do not do so. See https://www.health line.com/nutrition/oxalate-good-or-bad#section4 for more details.

Allowed Fruits

These fruits provide some burnable carbohydrates that keep your metabolism high, provides dietary fiber for your microbiome and provides energy while helping you avoid hunger.

Any reduced carbohydrate, non-tropical fruits with the exception that you may have grapefruit, lemons and limes if your doctor or pharmacist says it will not interfere with any prescriptions. Examples of these types of fruits are: apples, pears, peaches, plums, apricots, strawberries, blackberries, mulberries. You can continue the list with other similar tree fruits and berries. <u>Absolutely no</u> grapes, bananas, blueberries or date fruits.

Allowed Seafoods

Any non-predator fish unlimited. Predator fish only once a week due to mercury content. Try to get wild caught but don't worry if it is farm raised. Stay away from European and Asian farm raised[80]. White fish, sardines, smelts, salmon, tuna, trout, porgies, pollock, cod, catfish, snapper, mackerel, any fish with fins. Shrimp, lobster,

---

[80] It is all but impossible to stay away from Asian farm raised fish but always prefer North American farm raised as it is chemically cleaner.

crab, clams, oysters, abalone, most shellfish but limit scallops as they are very sweet. Squid, Octopus, molluscs and other seafoods of this type. No sea mammals.

Allowed Vegetables

These vegetables provide some carbohydrates, many nutrients and dietary fiber for your microbiome.

Lettuce, cabbage, celery, watercress, asparagus, bell peppers, cauliflower, string beans, mushrooms, okra, cucumbers, zucchini, konjac, radish, onions except not Sweet onions, Vidalia or Cipollini onions, most leafy green vegetables, including roasted seaweed, that are not sweet. There are many more. <u>Absolutely no</u> soybeans, tofu, corn, potatoes, beans, peas, beets, squash, carrots, plantains, parsnips or grains of any kind. Yes, that means no wheat, rye, barley, buckwheat or rice among others.

Other Not Allowed Foods

No tree nuts, peanuts, nuts or seeds of any kind. No corn, soy or liquid oils <u>other than</u> olive, A2 butter and coconut oil and those only in small quantities. No dairy of any kind.[81] No A1 butter, cheese, milk, cream,

---

[81] Except for type A2 Butter. Google it to learn more.

yogurt. No beer. No high sugar drinks, fruit juices, energy drinks, sodas or diet sodas.

Unlimited Foods

Any spice except for mixes that contain sugar or wheat. Salt, pepper, hot sauce, curries that do not contain wheat, vinegar, mustard.

Limited Quantity Foods

Mayonnaise, Thousand Island dressing (sugar free), Tartar Sauce, olive oil, coconut oil, any Asian based sauce that does not contain wheat and limit soy. (Look for soy free and/or wheat free soy sauce.) You can have Alabama style white BBQ sauce. It is best if you make your own mayonnaise using olive oil. Google "Blender Mayonnaise" and "heavy mayonnaise". If it tastes sweet don't eat it.   If you overeat mayonnaise, especially commercial mayonnaise which is made from poor quality oils you will not lose weight and might gain weight! You can also thin the mayonnaise with water, especially heavy mayonnaise which dilutes easier. Thinner mayonnaise coats everything better and at lower calorie costs!

Sweets

You can have any coffee flavoring if it does not contain sugar.

Cakes

You can eat all the Radatti Foods cakes and other products you want. I recently ate 2 cupcakes with sugar-free icing made of Radatti Foods High Fiber Cake Mix and I still lost a pound that day. www.radattifoods.com Try to not eat these cakes at night because that will give you a false weight reading in the morning. Drink water with all fiber-based products.

Alcohol Drinks and Water, Coffee, Tea

You may have 4oz (118 ml) of any dry wine per day. If you can avoid it, do so. No beer. Make sure you have the minimal doctor recommended amount of clear clean water per day. You may drink sparkling water, tea and coffee but no sodas of any kind. Try adding tea and/or lemon to sparkling water. Coffee and tea do not count as water so limit how much you drink.

General Directions

Keep a log of your weight on a daily or every other day basis. If you feel constipated mark that and do something about it. If you are not losing 1 pound every day you are doing something wrong or eating in excess or are constipated. Use a doctor approved laxative[82] or cut back on the fats depending upon the problem. If you significantly overeat for your metabolism or you do not keep to the schedule, you will not lose weight. The schedule is plus or minus 30 minutes. There are other issues that can cause you to not lose weight. Consult with a medical doctor. Eventually you will notice that you are eating less and less per meal. That is an indicator that your microbiome is moving in the correct direction. If this does not happen then stop eating before you are full and cut back a little bit every few days. You should notice that hunger goes away after about 30 to 40 minutes after eating. Never starve yourself but a little bit of a hunger edge is good.[83] If you are craving sweets just continue the diet, the craving

---

[82] I recently noticed that Castor Oil is once again available for constipation.

[83] "hara hachi bu"

https://www.huffpost.com/entry/not-overeating_b_96 9910

will go away as the bacteria in your microbiome that is causing the cravings die off.

Other details of this diet are under development. I am my own test subject as are friends. The full diet plan with lots of allowed high fiber treats will be published in a forthcoming book. Some of those treats will include safe all-natural calorie free sweeteners, cakes, cookies, bread and candies.

If you cheat on this diet do it with ketogenic approved foods and if you do not overeat it, you may still lose weight but at least not gain weight. Eventually you will reach a point where you are craving red meats. That is a good breaking point to go keto for a few weeks then back to the weight loss diet.

If you make a mistake forgive yourself and get back on the program! Be your own cheer leader.

Questions From Reviewers on Diet:

1. **I can never eat red meat?**
   Answer: This is a weight loss diet and is anti-inflammatory due to the natural fish oils. This is not and never was intended to be a lifelong diet. My guess is that it would be unhealthy to never eat red meats. Once you

reach your ideal weight go back to eating a healthy diet which includes red meats.

2. **Can I eat processed fish?**

   Answer: It depends. Certainly, you can eat canned/bottled fish and clams but check the ingredients to make sure there is nothing too harmful. Processed fish with stuffing from the market usually is full of grains and sugars which needs to be avoided. The same is true of processed crab cakes and fish cakes.

3. **I hate or am allergic to fish?**

   Answer: You can try to substitute organic, 100% pasture raised red meats and if it works, it works. Be careful if it says "pasture raised" that term is meaningless, only "100% pasture raised" has meaning. I make no promises other than fish worked for me.

4. **Is this diet healthy?**

   Answer: By definition no weight loss diet is healthy. You are doing body modification. The results may be good and the process may be worth the cost but the act of body modification induces physical stress which is never good. In addition, you medically may or may not be suitable for weight loss and should consult a medical doctor for the best answer.

5. How much should I weigh?

Answer: I am not a doctor and BMI[84] indexes are confusing. I suggest you start by talking with your medical doctor. For a historical perspective I will present the Metropolitan Life Insurance Company Desired Weights for Men and Women between the ages of 25 and 59 years from the year 1943. This chart was modified a few times after its introduction and assumed 1-inch heals on shoes. I corrected the chart to be bare footed. The charts also assume that you are wearing 5 pounds of clothing.

The company presented these charts prepared by Actuaries which indicates persons with the lowest mortality rates.

The 1943 charts were significant as being the first. Additional charts with changes were released in other years including 1959 and 1983.

I cannot tell you if these weights are still good and present them here for historical perspective only. Only a Medical Doctor can

---

[84] Body Mass Index

advise you on your individual and proper body weight.

<u>1943 Metropolitan Height Weight Chart</u>

<u>For Women</u> – Height in bare feet, Weight in pounds which includes 5 pounds of clothing. For nude -5.

Height Feet Inches	Small Frame	Medium Frame	Large Frame
4′ 9″	102-111	109-121	118-131
4′ 10″	103-113	111-123	120-134
4′ 11″	104-115	113-126	122-137
5′ 0″	106-118	115-129	125-140
5′ 1″	108-121	118-132	128-143
5′ 2″	111-124	121-135	131-147
5′ 3″	114-127	124-138	134-151
5′ 4″	117-130	127-141	137-155
5′ 5″	120-133	130-144	140-159
5′ 6″	123-136	133-147	143-163
5′ 7″	126-139	136-150	146-167
5′ 8″	129-142	139-153	149-170
5′ 9″	132-145	142-156	152-173
5′ 10″	135-148	145-159	155-176
5′ 11″	138-151	148-162	158-179

<u>1943 Metropolitan Height Weight Chart</u>

<u>For Men</u> – Height in bare feet, Weight in pounds which includes 5 pounds of clothing. For nude -5.

Height Feet Inches	Small Frame	Medium Frame	Large Frame
5′ 1″	128-134	131-141	138-150
5′ 2″	130-136	133-143	140-153
5′ 3″	132-138	135-145	142-156
5′ 4″	134-140	137-148	144-160
5′ 5″	136-142	139-151	146-164
5′ 6″	138-145	142-154	149-168
5′ 7″	140-148	145-157	152-172
5′ 8″	142-151	148-160	155-176
5′ 9″	144-154	151-163	158-180
5′ 10″	146-157	154-166	161-184
5′ 11″	149-160	157-170	164-188
6′ 0″	152-164	160-174	168-192
6′ 1″	155-168	164-178	172-197
6′ 2″	158-172	167-182	176-202
6′ 3″	162-176	171-187	181-207

Starter Recipes

Modified African Okro (Okra) Soup

(Fiber not Weight Loss – Maintenance Diet)

1. Shelled pumpkin seeds ½ cup. (available in most supermarkets)

2. Oxtail or stew beef. If you don't like beef use chicken or duck. Use about ½ pound.

3. Dried or smoked fish or shrimp or seafood of choice. Total 1 pound.

4. 3 cups of chopped green leafy vegetable.

5. Seasoning to taste: smoked paprika, red pepper flakes, salt.

6. Cut okra. Normally cut in rings but diced is good, 1 pound. Great source of dietary fiber!

7. Diced onions. ½ cup.

8. Fill with beef, chicken or duck bone broth.

Instructions

1. Medium soup pot, boil meat with seasoning, onions, pumpkin seeds for about 30 minutes or until done.

2. If fresh, wash and remove tops from okra then slice into rings. You can puree half of the okra if you desire. If frozen add to the pot at start.

3. After the contents of the pot is cooked add all the seafood. If the seafood is raw cook additional 5 minutes or until done. For defrosted fully cooked seafood cook an additional 2 minutes to warm.

4. Add all the remainder ingredients and cook until leaves are limp.

You can eat this right away, but left overs will improve overnight in the refrigerator.

Pete's Simple Cole Slaw

(Good for weight loss and fiber)

1. Using a food processor or good knife skills shred a small green cabbage.

2. Rinse the cabbage and drain until wet but not dripping.

3. Add mayonnaise[85] (google blender mayonnaise for healthy mayo using 100% olive and/or coconut oils) until everything is just coated but not clumpy. The water helps to coat everything without using excess mayo. You can also thin the mayonnaise with some water.

4. Add sea salt to taste and celery seeds / celery flakes if you have them.

5. Toss and refrigerate overnight.

Some people add sweeteners to Cole Slaw, but it does not need it. Cabbage is sweet on its own and no sweetener is needed. After a while, you will find commercial sweetened Cole Slaw disgusting.

---

[85] Heavy Mayonnaise has double egg yolks and tastes wonderful.

Pete's Simple Fish Cakes

(Good for weight loss)

1. Flake any inexpensive whitefish. This is easier to do if you bake the fish in the oven first. Make sure you fully debone the flakes as any bones can scratch or get caught in your mouth. You may want to run the flakes through a wire sieve if the fish has many small sharp bones.

2. Retain the scaled fish skin for making fish skin Chicharrons. You can freeze them for later.

3. Add egg to the fish flakes. If you want extra rich use duck eggs. Mix until moist but not dripping. Add more egg or fish flakes as needed.

4. Season. You can add Old Bay seasoning but be careful it can get salty tasting if you over use it. Alternately, my favorite is to add flaked dried parsley, basil, onion flakes, celery seeds, pinch of sea salt and cracked black pepper. You can add garlic or onion powered if you desire. In fact, you can add almost any seasoning you like including hot sauce.

5. Make small balls and flatten into cakes about the size of a silver dollar pancake.

6. Pan fry preferably on a cast iron skillet with a tiny amount of olive oil for taste.

7. Refrigerate.

Three fish cakes make a very filling meal.

Fish Skin Chicharrons

(Good for weight loss)

This is a very tasty Asian dish. People in the west are used to Chicharrons and fish skins sound odd even though we already eat them. Think crunchy "Salmon Skin Roll". I modified this from a fried dish to a broiled dish for diet purposes.

1. Wash fish skin. Make sure all scales are removed and the skin looks fresh and clean. Smell test them.

2. Put them in a bag and add a small amount of melted coconut oil to just coat the skins. Shake.

3. In a well-ventilated room put the skins on a roasting pan and set on a high rack in hot oven. Set oven to broil. You can use a flat iron weight if you want them to be perfectly flat. You can also pan fry them if you use the iron.

4. Watch carefully the skins burn easily and will not be eatable. The skins will shrink and curl. Turn once. Remove quickly when completely cooked and eat at room temperature.

Like all fish, this dish can spoil quickly so be sure to refrigerate any left overs and dispose of as soon as they look, smell or taste "funny".

This is a hard dish to make but rewarding if you get it right. Think guilt free crunchy snack! Most people who make this fry them, but we don't want all the extra fat. Google "fish skin chicharrons" for more ideas.

You can experiment with the flavors you add to the fish skins. Try onion powder. You may find this hard to believe but google "salty egg fish skins". It is a popular snack food and is made commercially. I like them.

Chia Seed Pudding

(Good for weight loss and dietary fiber)

Two tablespoons of Chia Seeds contain 10 grams of fiber in addition to omega 3 fatty acids that fight inflammation.

There are many recipes on the Internet for chia seed puddings. Look at them, then my recipe and decide what you want.

1. In a coffee cup of hot water add 3 rounded tablespoons of Coffee Mate or other non-dairy coffee creamer. Different people may like more or less. You can use Almond Milk, Coconut Milk or Cashew Milk but they will contain a lot more calories and fats.

2. Add the hot fake-milk to a large jar with a lid. Add enough room temperature water to total 2 cups of combined milk and water.

3. Add any allowed sweetener and flavoring. Do not use sugar of any type. My favorites are vanilla, mango and coconut.

4. Add 6 rounded tablespoons of chia seeds and stir. Put on the lid and refrigerate. The next day

it will be ready. If too thin add more Chia seeds and put back in refrigerator. You may need to stir again.

Keep for 1 week or more in a cold refrigerator.

Chia seed pudding can cause constipation so don't over eat. When you eat this be sure to drink water at the same time to assist proper digestion. Never eat dry chia seeds as that can cause serious medical problems.

Pete's Tartar Sauce

(small amounts ok for weight loss – no fiber)

I love tartar sauce. I know a lot of people hate anything mayonnaise based but I don't. I do however really dislike commercial tartar sauce which has lots of unnecessary sugar which destroys the taste of the sauce. For that reason, I have been making my own for as long as I can remember.

A lot of my recipes are "by hand" that means I make things by feel and look. There are no recipes. For that reason and because everyone likes things a little different, I am going to give you the basic recipe and you modify it according to your taste.

½ cup of mayonnaise. (Heavy Mayo is wonderful[86])
1 tablespoon sweet pickle relish
1 teaspoon of lemon juice.
Optional: Add water to thin out. You will use less.

Mix well and enjoy. Do not over eat!

---

[86] Heavy Mayonnaise has double the egg yolks. Google for details.

Pete's Japanese Style Tartar Sauce

Take the tartar sauce from above and add either a very small amount of Wasabi[87] or standard American horseradish. American horseradish is usually in a light vinegar base. I prefer the American horseradish. One of the reasons is that fresh Wasabi tastes very different from the powders and pastes that are easy to get in the United States, while American horseradish is always consistent.

---

[87] A green very strong horse radish. Please note, **very strong!**

Pete's Italian Seasoning Mix

(good for weight loss and fiber)

People seem to think that Italian mix should have a strong oregano and garlic taste but that is far from the truth. Oregano is only used as an after-taste in real northern Italian cooking. Garlic can be a front or an after-taste but never dominate. If you were eating a roasted garlic rosemary chicken it should taste like chicken first, then rosemary and garlic second. This is my family recipe which has been in use for 2 or 3 generations.

Equal weights of Basil and Parsley. Mix in a bowel and crush between your hands until everything is a consistence size and mix.

That's it and you won't get finer.

How to Buy Garlic and Onion Powder

(good for weight loss and fiber)

Everyone wants to sell you garlic salt and onion salt. That stuff is low quality. Is salt hard to find? No. The salt in these mixes are to take up space and because they can use lower quality powders. It is also low-end salt. Only buy pure garlic powder and onion powder. Garlic powder is easy to find but if you can't find onion powder look for "Cebolla en polvo". It is the same thing but is the Mexican name for onion powder. Granulated and powder is not the same thing.

One of the things you can do with the onion powder is to sprinkle it on cooked fish. If you sprinkle it heavy it will almost take on the texture of a breading coat but not be overpowering in flavor.

Pete's Chinese Style String Beans

(good for weight loss and fiber)

Chinese style string beans are usually cooked in a fryolator in restaurants. I don't own one, so I use a deep-frying pan with only a light coating of oil. Buy precut skinny string beans. They are sometimes called Extra Fine Green Beans. I have also heard them called French String Beans.

Toss the beans with enough olive or coconut oil so they are all coated but not drippy. Put them in the frying pan on high heat. Only do a small amount at one time. As soon as they start to look a little wrinkly take then out, sprinkle salt, onion and/or garlic powder. They will finish cooking on the plate. You want them a little crunchy.

This is not authentic Chinese which is why I call them Chinese Style.

Pakistani Style Curry Cauliflower

(good for weight loss and fiber)

A good friend taught me this dish. Until you taste this you won't believe how wonderful it is. There is a secret which is to use Pakistani Curry and not Indian Curry. There are large differences in flavor and how they are used. Indian curry usually contains wheat and is used for sauce. Pakistani curry is pure herbals and is used dry.

In a deep-frying pan break an entire head of cauliflower into fleurettes. Also break up and use the stem. I differ from the real thing here in that I add water and cover the pan for 10 minutes or until the cauliflower can be easily pierced with a fork. DO NOT OVERCOOK. I used to hate cauliflower but that is because it was always served as an over boiled mush. This stuff if fantastic.

Now for the secret ingredient. Buy "Shan" brand Vegetable Masala. It is pure and flavorful. I buy it from amazon.com. Not only is this inexpensive but because it is pure it lasts a lot longer than you might think.

Make sure the cauliflower is dry in the hot pan. Start to sprinkle the Shan Masala on the cauliflower while continuing to stir the pan. Do not stop stirring. When everything has a golden color, taste it. Add more if you want. Remember you can always add more but it's hard to remove. As soon as everything is coated remove from heat and plate it. Eat hot or cold.

When I told you, my secret is "Shan" Vegetable Masala it really is. I use it on fish, chicken, red meats and all kinds of vegetables. Shan also makes a bunch of other curries all equally good, but I found the Vegetable Masala very versatile.

Pete's Foies (Verza Stufata) Diet Version

(good for weight loss and fiber)

I have only known this dish as Foies or Foyes. I can't find it on the Internet by that name, but the secondary name appears to be close enough. This is a lightly flavored sweet dish thanks to the Savoy cabbage. I never found anyone who disliked it. The cabbage contributes Vitamin K (40.17%), Vitamin C (24.11%), Vitamin B9 (14.00%), Vitamin B6 (10.23%) and dietary Fiber (5.79%) per cup.

> 1 full sized head of Savoy cabbage (Must use Savoy)
> 4 gloves of fresh garlic
> ½ cup of yellow virgin olive oil.

1) Tear cabbage by hand and tear each leaf into fork sized pieces. Don't forget about shrinkage.
2) Boil slightly salted water then add the cabbage.
3) Boil cabbage for about half an hour until tender but not mushy. You will want to remove it a little early.
4) As soon as the cabbage is done remove from stove and drain most but not all the water. Leaving some water is important.   Everything will continue to cook so be careful not to overcook.

5) Before you are done boiling the cabbage, using a deep-frying pan add all the olive oil and the cloves of garlic. Bring to heat and toss the garlic until they are dark walnut colored and soft.

6) As soon as done, pour the oil and garlic over the cabbage, quickly add salt to taste and gently toss. It will make a sizzling sound and be careful of splatter! The oil is a critical flavor component. Please be aware that many brands, including imported brands, of olive oil in the United States and Canada are fake or low grade being passed off as high grade. Costco brand olive oil is high quality.

7) If the garlic is not strong enough add powdered garlic and/or more salt.

8) Let sit for at least 10 minutes then enjoy!

You can add fish, shrimp or any seafood to this dish, but I tend to eat it as is.

This dish will taste even better the next day. Refrigerate remainders for up to 1 week depending upon your refrigerator. In my family we often eat this as the main dish.

The non-diet version of this dish adds potatoes and/or smoked ham.

My uncle likes to keep more water than I usually do. It makes it a bit soupy which I also like. The water picks up the flavors and makes a vegetable broth.

Greco-Roman Salad Dressing Mix

There is no standard formula for this dressing. It was given to me by the chief at a Greco-Roman restaurant in Suffern New York. Just play around with the amounts until you like the flavor.

Garlic – fresh minced or powdered

Lemon juice with some grated rind

Fresh or dry basil.

Salt

Black or white pepper.

Oregano

You can use this dry on damp salad or mix it with olive oil. You can also use it as a dry mix on fish or seafood. Experiment by adding onion powder or other seasonings. Do not over use the oil.

The salad in New York included lettuce and lots of seafoods such as shrimp and squid.

Pete's General Advise on Diet Foods

The reason so many people drop a diet is because it becomes boring. There is no reason for any diet to become boring. Seasoning, herbs, sauces and different cooking styles all exist that make food look, smell and taste different. You can eat the exact same dish every day for months and have it taste different every time. Most people only eat fried fish. You can but you have to fry it without the breading in 1 teaspoon of oil. You can "bread" it afterward with onion powder. You have never tasted fish until you BBQ grilled it on a smoky fire. Buy wood chips for your BBQ (works even with gas) and each wood will give the fish a different flavor and color. I cook on a $20 cast-iron charcoal hibachi and that works great.

I found I love the taste of fully cooked but room temperature or even cold fish. It has a sweet taste. The same is true of the fish cakes. I bring them to work and eat them at room temperature.

Here are a few flavors (all available on amazon.com) you can try that are on the weight loss diet:

Butcher's Black Pepper – A very different and wonderful flavor from the stuff you are used to.

Salad dressing – Take any mayo-based salad dressing and thin it out with water. You can easily replace 25% with water and it will taste just as good, spreads better and has only 75% of the calories. Put on fish or vegetables and of course salad. Do not over eat!

Mustard – Not the yellow paste you are used to. Buy Stone Ground Mustard! Here is what should be in it: Water, Mustard Seed, vinegar, salt, citric acid, turmeric. It has a flavor that is much more robust than usual, and you can water it down or mix it with mayo to make sauces for fish or vegetables.

BBQ Sauce – Most BBQ sauces are mostly sugar but there are a few that are not. My favorite is Northern Alabama Style BBQ sauce. There are two brands I like, "Big Bob Gibson Bar-B-Q Original White Sauce" and "Lillie's Q Barbeque Sauce IVORY". These are great on fish, chicken and vegetables including salad.

Asian Style Sauces – There are more Asian sauces than you could taste in a life time. I want you to stay gluten free so there is a brand that I found that tastes good and I still lose weight on it. San-J brand is gluten free. www.san-j.com for details and recipes. There is sugar in these sauces but not enough that it will stop weight loss. The sauces are thin and spread. They are very flavorful and give a great kick to everything.

Hot Sauces – There are more hot sauces in the world than I could count. Most of them are not very good being all heat and no flavor. There is one hot sauce that dominates the southern United States and that is Crystal.   At this point you can find it in supermarkets in the northern states. This stuff is good. www.baumerfoods.com

Mayonnaise – Take mayonnaise and replace 25% with water. It becomes a thin tasty sauce that is great on salad, vegetables and fish. Flavor it with lemon, lime juices, garlic powder, etc.

Lemons & Limes – Why do people always forget that lemons and limes taste so good on fish, vegetables and salad? This stuff is great, and they taste very different. You can also combine them to make a lemon-lime flavor like the soda.

Himalayan Pink Salt – This tastes better than sea salt or table salt. There are many different types of salts that all taste different. Try Black Salt for an eggy/sulfur surprise. Indian kitchens usually carry several salts for the family cook.

Wakame – Wakame roasted seaweed comes in wafers, salads and shredded. I love the wafers which can be eaten with fish or as a snack. The salad often has sugar added so make your own.

Referenced Books and Films

Books

"Dietary Fiber, Essential to the Human Microbiome and Health"
by Peter V. Radatti.
ISBN-13: 978-1545015421

"The Big Fat Surprise: Why Butter, Meat and Cheese Belong in a Healthy Diet"
by Nina Teicholz
ISBN-13: 978-1451624434

"Pure, White, and Deadly: How Sugar Is Killing Us and What We Can Do to Stop It"
by Doctor John Yudkin
ISBN-13: 978-0143125181

"How the Ideology of Low Fat Conquered America"

by Ann F. La Berge.

Journal of the History of Medicine and Allied Sciences, Volume 63, Issue 2, 1 April 2008, Pages 139–177, https://doi.org/10.1093/jhmas/jrn001
Published: 23 February 2008
https://academic.oup.com/jhmas/article/63/2/139/772615

Films

Both films are available on www.amazon.com

"That Sugar Movie" by Damon Gameau.

http://Samuelgoldwynfilms.com
http://thatsugarfilm.com

"The Magic Pill" by Pete Evans

Gravitas Ventures   www.peteevans.com

Great Videos on Gut Brain Connection:

"Science Nature Page" by Hashem Al-Ghaili

https://www.facebook.com/ScienceNaturePage/videos/480707825745279/

and

https://www.facebook.com/watch/?query=gut%20brain

<u>Other Books That I Am Reading</u>

This is a list of a few of the books that I decided to share. This is not an endorsement of the books, their contents or authors. It is only a list of what I am reading.

"Vitamin K2 and the Calcium Paradox"

Kate Rheaume-Bleue, B.Sc., N.D.

Extract from the back cover:

Are you taking calcium or vitamin D? This book could save your life!

Learn the secret to avoiding osteoporosis and heart disease. Millions of people take vitamin D and calcium supplements for bone health. But new research shows that this actually increases the risk of heart attack and stroke because extra calcium builds up in the arteries – the Calcium Paradox. The secret to keeping bones strong and arteries clear is vitamin K2, a little-known super-nutrient that humans once consumed in abundance and that has been ignored by scientists for almost 70 years.

Peter V. Radatti

"The Magnesium Miracle"

Carolyn Dean, M.D., N.D.

Extract from the back cover:

Magnesium is an essential nutrient, indispensable to your health and well-being. By adding this mineral to your diet, you are guarding against – and helping to alleviate – such threats as heart disease, stroke, osteoporosis, diabetes, depression, arthritis, and asthma. But despite magnesium's numerous benefits, many Americans remain dangerously deficient.

<u>My Favorite Prebiotics</u>
<u>and Probiotics</u>

GrainFields

There are a lot of brands of probiotics on the market. I feel that, at one time or another, I have purchased all of them. Very few seem to have any detectable effect on me. The expensive ones had the same effect as the inexpensive ones; nothing.

While visiting my distributor in Brooklyn, they handed me a bottle of Grainfields probiotic liquid. They import it from Australia. I did not expect much, but it had a noticeable benefit. When I gave it to elderly relatives, it had a pronounced beneficial effect. While I have not used probiotics daily, I now have a favorite and it is Grainfields.

Grainfields is made from a blend of malt, oats, maize, rice, wheat, millet and buckwheat. I don't like using grains that contain gluten, but I was unofficially told that the gluten is digested by the bacteria and would qualify as gluten-free, if they could afford the costs of making that legal claim. I am gluten-intolerant and have not experienced any problems using the product. However, buyer beware. Decide for yourself or ask your medical doctor.

The bacteria Grainfields uses to make their product are certified organic, non-GMO, and non-Genetically Modified. They claim that the strains used are all present in a healthy, human digestive system and are, therefore, good for anyone who is missing these strains. The strains used are:

- Lactobacillus Acidophilus

- Bifidus (Bifidobacterium)

- Lactobacillus casi

- Lactobacillus helveticus

- Lactobacillus bulgaricus

- Lactobacillus leichmannii

- Lactobacillus caucasicus

- Lactobacillus lactis

- Lactobacillus fermenti

- Lactobacillus brevis

- Lactobacillus plantarum

- Lactobacillus delbreukii

with healthy yeast strains:

- Saccharomyces boulardi

- Saccharomyces cerevisiae.

One of the reasons why I believe that some of the probiotics I've used in the past had no effect is because the stomach acid probably killed the bacteria before they could work. The yeasts used in this product are proven to be acid-resistant and are known to provide beneficial enzymes and B vitamins as a by-product, in addition to their ability to kill Candida. Candida infections can be common.

www.grainfieldsusa.com
Grainfields USA LLC /The Essence of Life®
451 6th Ave. Brooklyn, NY. 11215

Grainfields@icloud.com OR r.grainfieldsusa@gmail.com
Phone: 1-718-788-8783   Cell 347-236-6334

Wholesale inquiries welcome ~ Rebecca Grainfields

Mother Dirt

I learned about the microbiome of the skin from a book which discussed a product from a company called Mother Dirt. This fit right in with my thirst for knowledge about the microbiome of the entire body. It also fit with some of my past experiences. I once met a doctor from Bulgaria. She was a Doctor of Cosmetology. I told her that I didn't understand her title because a Cosmetologist was a title in the United States, but it was someone who sold cosmetics. She was shocked and went on to explain what she did. Her profession is a medical doctor who diagnoses a patient by looking at them. She is especially careful to examine the skin because "all the problems of the body are exhibited on the skin". What she does is like what a family doctor does in the United States but, because they don't have all the fancy diagnostic equipment, they use a different paradigm.

This made me think, if the outside reflects the inside, then does the outside affect the inside? Is it a two-way street? Can improvement of our skin's health affect our internal health? This is yet to be proven, but I would be surprised if it is not true.

This experience made me instantly understand the importance of the microbiome of the skin and what the Mother Dirt company is attempting to do, which is nothing short of correcting the skin microbiome with direct application of one specific bacterium that makes the skin a much healthier (and beautiful) place for beneficial bacteria to grow, while suppressing bad or imbalanced bacteria.

I purchase a single bottle of the Mother Dirt product "AO+MIST" and was so impressed that I purchased a subscription for 1 bottle every 3 months. As I continued to use the product and saw the benefits for myself, I expanded the use of the product and changed my subscription from 1 bottle every 3 months to 1 bottle every 2 months.

Here is information from the label of the bottle:

> INGREDIENTS: Water, Nitrosomonas Eutropha (live, cultured, Ammonia-Oxidizing Bacteria), disodium phosphate, magnesium chloride (natural salts). FOR TOPICAL USE ONLY.

They continue with an explanation of the product:

> Formulated for compatibility with the skin's natural microbiome. Learn more at biomefriendly.com.
> Questions: hello@motherdirt.com

Their website is www.motherdirt.com

Radatti Foods, LLC

This is the company that I own. As of this writing we expect to be in production Summer 2019. Everything that this company will produce will be microbiome friendly, high fiber – healthy fats and always low insulin response.
www.radattifoods.com

You will have to check the website for details on when and where products will be made available.

<u>Glossary</u>[88]

<u>A</u>

Acetate—derivative of acetic acid. Used as a counter-irritant and a reagent in chemical reactions.

ADA—Americans with Disabilities Act regulates compliance with regulations protecting the disabled.

Alanine Aminotransferase (ALT) enzymes—an enzyme that converts amino acid L-Alanine to L-glutamate

Alimentary—organ system that includes the mouth, esophagus, stomach, intestines, and anus, used to digest food and eliminate wastes from the body.

Amylose—a polysaccharide chain that is found in some starches

Anaphylactic—acute, unhealthy reaction to a substance that was previously encountered. Reactions can range from mere itching to shock and death.

---

[88] Courtesy of http://www.online-medical-dictionary.org/ and http://medical-dictionary.thefreedictionary.com/ and http://en.wikipedia.org/wiki/

Antimicrobial agents—any substance that can destroy or prevent spread of microbes

Apnea—absence of breathing, especially during sleep.

Aspartame—artificial sweetener, irritates nervous system and stomach lining, alters gut flora

ATP—a neurotransmitter, also an energy-transfer molecule in the cell

Atherosclerosis—so-called "hardening of the arteries" by fat deposits on blood vessel walls

Autoimmune—body's immune system begins to attack the tissues of the body for no discernible reason.

B

Bacteria—one-celled organisms, can be either beneficial or malignant to the human body

Bacillus coagulans—a beneficial bacteria found in the gut, rarely pathogenic, aids with food digestion.

BHA/BHT—food additive that is an endocrine disruptor

Bifidobacterium-- infantis, animalis, breve, bifidum—beneficial bacteria found in the gut, aids with food digestion.

Bile—created by the liver, it assists in digestion of fats in the duodenum.

Biomarker—something biological used to identify or measure its presence in another substance

BMI—Basal Metabolic Index—a measure of body fat based on height/weight.

Butyrate—a short-chain fatty acid used in flavoring extracts and perfumes

<u>C</u>

Candida—yeast-like fungus normally found in alimentary canal, but can overgrow and cause problems

Carbohydrate—a combination of carbon, hydrogen, and oxygen; a food source of energy for the body, such as sugars and starches. Can be changed into fats in large quantities. Polysaccharides are also carbs.

Cardiovascular—pertaining to the heart and its blood vessels.

Cellulose—carbohydrates that form the structures of plants. Polysaccharide. Dietary fiber.

Chitin—a polysaccharide that makes up insect shells and certain fungi. Like cellulose.

Cholesterol—found in animal fats and oils, that makes up most of the body cell walls, can create stones. Usually created by the body's liver.

Circadian rhythm—cycle between day and night. A 24-hour cycle

Colonocytes—the inside-most cell of the lining of the large intestine.

Clostridium difficile—bacteria found in human feces. Can cause illness if it infects other organs or in case of overgrowth.

Colon—the large intestine of the human alimentary canal. Aids in digestion and re-absorption of water from stool.

Colitis—inflammation of the large intestine due to infection or overgrowth of bacteria. May cause diarrhea, cramping, and pain.

Constipation—an inability to pass stool due to low motility, or blockage, of the large intestine/sigmoid colon/rectum.

Contrabiotic--blocks mucosal adherence and relocation of bad bacteria in the colon and may diminish intestinal inflammation,

Cristae-- folds on the inside wall of the mitochondria

Crohn's Diseases—form of chronic inflammation involving the distal small and complete large intestine, with ulcers, narrowing of the passage, and flu-like symptoms.

Cruciferous vegetables—broccoli, cabbage, and other green, leafy vegetables, part of the mustard family

Cytoplasm—gel-like substance inside cell walls, also called protoplasm. Contains organelles like mitochondria.

D

Dendritic cell—a branch of a nerve cell that carries impulses to another place.

Diverticulitis—inflammation of a pocket in the intestine (diverticulum) that may cause pain and rupture if filled with feces.

Disaccharides—sugar created by two monosaccharides, such as lactose or sucrose.

DNA—genetic material that acts as the blueprint for reproduction of a cell.

Duodenal Ulcer—an inflammatory ulcer of the mucous membrane in the high small intestine.

Dysbiosis—unhealthy, unbalanced biome, such as when antibiotics are used.

<u>E</u>

Endogenous—internally produced by an organism, tissue, or cell

Enzyme—a compound that serve to initiate a biochemical reaction.

F

Fauna—animal life, includes microbes.

Fiber, water-insoluble—fiber that doesn't dissolve in water and maintains its original properties.

Fiber, water-soluble—fiber that dissolves in water and becomes gel-like

Fecal transplant—transplant of healthy fecal matter from one human gut biome to another

Feces—waste matter of the body, made up of dead microbes, fiber, undigested food, dead cells

Fibromyalgia—inflammatory disorder of the nervous and muscle tissues, causing pain, stiffness.

Flatulence—gaseous by-products of digestion, emitted by the anus.

Flora—vegetable life, including fungi and yeast

Fructans—polymer of fructose molecules

Fructo-oligosaccharide—fructan with a short chain length

Fungicide—a substance that kills fungi or fungal spores

G

Gastroesophageal reflux—the weakening of the cardiac sphincter of the stomach, allowing gastric contents to move up the esophagus under pressure

Gastrointestinal—pertaining to the stomach and intestinal tract

Gelatin—a solution of soluble fiber and water

Gestational Diabetes—type II diabetes that occurs because of pregnancy; may be temporary.

Glucose—single sugar, used as fuel for all tissues of the body.

Glycoside—plant-derived component of a drug or poison

Glyphosate—RoundUp, a pesticide that can alter the gut microbiome, found on plants

GMO—Genetically Modified Organism.

Goodbelly—a probiotic drink containing lactobacillus plantarum

Grainfields—probiotic supplement, provides yeast for microbiome growth

Gut—collective of stomach, intestines, sigmoid colon, & rectum.

H

Helminths—worms. Some, such as hookworms, tapeworms, and whipworms, can be beneficial to the gut biome. Others are parasitic.

Hemicellulose—polysacchaarides which make up the cell walls of plants.

Herbicides—chemical substances that kill plants.

Herbivores—plant-eating animals.

Hexose—simple sugars containing six carbon atoms, such as glucose and fructose.

HFCS—High Fructose Corn Syrup. Contains glucose and fructose polymers. A high-caloric sweetener

HFS—A high-caloric sweeter like HFCS.

Hyperglycemia—elevated level of sugar in the blood, usually found in diabetes mellitus

Hypertension—persistently elevated blood pressure, usually above 140/100.

I

Immune-modulating—natural, non-allergic substances that support the immune system.

Immunoglogulin E—Antibody found in mammals, fights parasites.

Inositol—multiple-alcohol sugar

Inflammation----immune response of the body to attacking organisms. Redness, heat, pain, itching may be part of the response.

TNF-a—tumor necrosis factor alpha, a protein involved in acute inflammation reaction

Insulin resistance—condition in which pancreatic cells don't respond to the hormone insulin, resulting in hyperglycemia.

Inulin—a natural carbohydrate that stores sugar in the body.

Irritable Bowel Syndrome—a group of symptoms indicating irritation in bowel, including pain, change in bowel habits, cramping. There is no apparent disease process.

Isoflavones—also called phytoestrogens. Estragenic-like substance found in plants.

K

Kombucha—fermented, slightly carbonated black or green tea drink. Produced by fermenting tea using beneficial bacteria and yeast

L

Lactobacillus-- plantarum, acidophilus, rhamnosus, paracasei, casei, fermentum—a form of bacteria that converts sugar to lactic acid in the gut.

Lactulose—non-absorbable sugar used for constipation and to treat liver toxicity

Laparoscopic—examination of the inside of the abdomen using a thin viewing device called a laparoscope.

Leaky gut—a condition of increased permeability (leaking) of the intestinal wall, causing inflammation throughout the body.

Leukocytes—cells of the immune system that protect against disease and parasites.

Lignan—one of the phytoestrogens that also acts as an antioxidant... usually found in nut, seeds, grains, some beans and fruits, and cruciferous vegetables.

LPS-induced inflammation—lipopolysaccharides found in tobacco and some dusts can cause inflammation and damage in the respiratory system.

<u>M</u>

Metabolic syndrome—a cluster of symptoms that are associated with cardiovascular disease and type II Diabetes. They include obesity, high blood pressure and serum triglycerides and low high- density lipoprotein.

Microbes—a microscopic organism, may be single-celled or a colony

Microbiome—the flora and fauna of a particular system; in this case, the gut of a human being

Monoshccharides—simple sugars, most basic carbohydrate. Used to build more complex sugars. Glucose, fructose, galactose are simple sugars.

Monomeric—single-named.

MRSA-- methicillin-resistant Staphylococcus aureus—a microbe found mostly in soil and are different from S. Aureus. Resistant to penicillin-related antibiotics. May be fatal.

MSG—a flavoring agent, also a neurotoxin

Mucosa—mucous membrane, lining the nose, mouth, eyes, and genitals.

Myocardial infarction—commonly known as a "heart attack"; damage done to the heart from a blocked vessel.

<u>N</u>

Necrotizing enterocolitis—severe inflammation of the small and large intestines, leading to death of tissue.

Neurogastroenterology—the study of the interactions of the brain, nervous system, and the gut.

Neurological—relating to the nervous system.

Neurons—cells in the nervous system that transmit electrical impulses throughout the body

O

Obesity—excess body fat which may have an adverse effect on health as determined by BMI

Occam's razor—Theory that "the simplest explanation is usually the best."

Oligosaccharides—a sugar polymer containing a small number of simple sugars.

P

Pathogenic—injurious to health

Pectin—a structural polysaccharide found in the cell walls of plants. A dietary fiber.

Pentose—a sugar containing 5 carbon atoms, such as ribose and xylose.

Pesticides—chemical substances that kill "pests", such as weeds, insects, worms, rats, mice, microbes, etc.

Phytic acid—the principle storage form of phosphorus in bran, seeds, cereals, and grains.

Platelets—a blood cell that stops bleeding by clotting off injured blood vessel walls.

Polydextrose—synthetic polymer of glucose; a soluble fiber.

Polymer—a large molecule made up of many repeating sub-units bound together to create things like plastics and resins.

Polysaccharide—a carbohydrate made up of long chains of simple sugars.

Polyuronides—a polysaccharide made up of uronic acid molecules, may have other simple sugars or not.

Prebiotic—substances that promote the growth or activity of beneficial microbes

Probiotic—microbes that claim to provide health benefits

Preservatives—chemical that lengthens the shelf life of products by preventing decomposition of its components.

Propionate—common short-chain fatty acid produced by the gut in response to indigestible fiber.

Pseudomonas aeruginosa—a multi-drug-resistant pathogen that attacks during other illnesses.

R

rBGT—recombinant Bovine Growth Hormone—a diabetogenic hormone, with links to cancer. It promotes milk production in cows.

Resistant starch—R1, R2, R3 are fermented by the gut microbiota, which produce short-chain fatty acids.

Rheumatological—pertaining to rheumatic diseases, usually of the joints and bones.

Rhinovirus—common cold virus. "rhino" refers to the nose.

Ribosomes—organelles in the cell that are responsible for protein synthesis.

RNA—a polymer required to code, decode, regulate, and express genes in the cell.

Roughage—insoluble fiber.

<u>S</u>

Saccharide—a sugar molecule

Salmonella—enterobacterium that causes vomiting and diarrhea when ingested. Found in poorly-stored food. Also known as "food poisoning"

SCFA--Short Chain Fatty Acids--fatty acids with 2-6 carbon atoms. Also referred to as "volatile fatty acids"

SHBG--Sex Hormone Binding Globulin--a glycoprotein that binds to androgen and estrogen.

Slippery elm—the "slippery" inner bark of the tree is used as a fiber to regulate the bowels.

Sodium nitrate/nitrite—food preservative that causes cancer

Streptococcus thermophilus—a lactic-acid microbe that ferments milk products.

Sucralose—artificial sweetener, irritates the nervous system and stomach lining and alters gut flora

Symbiotes—symbiotic bacteria that live with other organisms to their mutual advantage.

T

T-cell—a type of white blood cell that assists in cell-mediated immunity.

Toxins—a poison or venom of plant or animal origin which causes disease when present in low doses.

V

Vaginosis—inflammation of the vagina due to overgrowth of bacteria, with foul odor, discharge, itching.

Vitamin D—fat-soluble vitamin that assist in absorption of calcium and other vital minerals.

Vitamin K—fat-soluble vitamin that is responsible for blood clotting and assists with calcium management.

Additional Books by Peter V. Radatti

www.radatti.com/books

A Fun Short Course in Beginning Radionics
43 pages, September 2013, ASIN B00EZTBRGI
Kindle only.

A Fun Course in Beginning Radionics Third Edition
394 pages, January 2017, ISBN-13: 978-1542419970

Un curso divertido de iniciacion a la RADIONICA: Milagros en las palmas de tus manos
Spanish language very of Radionics book.
270 pages, November 2018, ISBN-13: 978-1726465458

How to Build an Electronic Witness Well for Radionics
44 pages, June 2017, ISBN-13: 978-1545124819

Dietary Fiber: Essential To The Human Microbiome and Health
118 pages, June 2018, ISBN-13: 978-1545015421

Peter V. Radatti

Fibra Dietetica: Esencial Para El Microbioma Humano Y La Salud

124 pages, August 2018, ISBN-13: 978-1725715660

VFind Security Tool Kit Handbook (5th Edition): Unix/Linux Computer Security

344 pages, December 2014, ISBN-13: 978-1533465139

Why Would I Want to Be an Ant?

79 pages, January 31, 2019, ISBN: 9781790544141

Reader's Notes